CONTENTS

INTRODUCTION

Changes in the lifestyle and dietary habits over the last decades have resulted in an "outbreak" of a worldwide pandemic of obesity that shortens the lifespans of the affected individuals, and together with the associated metabolic complications, constitute a significant socioeconomic problem. Obesity, especially when associated with the accumulation of visceral adipose tissue, shortens lifespan indirectly by increasing the risk of developing many diseases, including hypertension, type 2 diabetes mellitus (T2DM), and hyperlipidemia—major components of metabolic syndrome. Apart from the strictly medical aspects, the growing prevalence of obesity is a significant socio-economic problem. It has been shown that obesity negatively affects personal and working relations and it is estimated that treatment of overweight and obese individuals' costs, on average, 30%–40% more than health care for people of normal weight .

Major goals in the treatment of obesity include not only weight reduction, but also a reduction of obesity-related complications such as insulin-resistance, hyperlipidemia and cardiovascular diseases. The most commonly used method of treating obesity is calorie restriction (CR) combined with increased physical activity; bariatric surgery, which is effective but also the most expensive, efficacy of other medical therapies is limited and therefore there is a constant need for novel, non-invasive methods for the treatment of obesity and related complications.

In the research on the pathogenesis and consequences of obesity, a state of permanent over-nutrition, studies on CR have been particularly helpful. These studies identified sirtuins (silent information regulators, SIRTs) as important players in different cellular metabolic pathways and seem to be interesting therapeutic targets in the treatment of obesity and related complications. SIRTs' activities are not limited to the metabolism regulation and include, among others, control of longevity, oncogenesis as well as neurological and cardiovascular functions.

CHAPTER 1 : Short Review of the Silent Information Regulators (SIRTs) System

The SIRTs comprise of a family of highly conserved regulatory proteins present in virtually all species. Originally, SIRTs were identified as class III histone deacetylases, nicotinamide adenine dinucleotide (NAD) dependent enzymes responsible for the removal of acetyl groups from lysine residues in proteins; however, some members of this family also act as mono-ADP-ribosyltransferases. Acetylation and deacetylation is an important mechanism of posttranslational modifications responsible for protein activation or inactivation and therefore, for the regulation of distinct cellular pathways. Indeed, the list of SIRTs targets in mammals includes, among others, those involved in the regulation of cell survival, apoptosis, inflammatory and stress responses, as well as lipid and glucose homeostasis.

In mammals, seven SIRT genes (SIRTs) have been identified that encode seven distinct SIRT enzymes of different structure, cellular localization, and tissue expression. Despite variable length and sequence, all SIRTs have a highly conserved catalytic core region consisting of approximately 275 amino acids, forming a Rossmann-fold domain (characteristic of NAD+/NADH binding proteins) and a zinc-binding domain connected by several loops. Outside the catalytic core, SIRT enzymes possess variable N- and C-terminal regions that determine their enzymatic activities, binding partners and substrates, as well as subcellular localization. SIRT1, SIRT6 and SIRT7 are predominantly found in the nucleus where via modifications of transcription factors, cofactors and histones they participate in the regulation of energy metabolism, stress and inflammatory responses, DNA repair (SIRT1 and SIRT6), and rDNA transcription (SIRT7). SIRT2 is present in the cytoplasm and primarily plays a role in cell cycle control. SIRT3 is located in mitochondria and takes part in the regulation of metabolic enzymes (e.g., those involved in glycolysis, fatty acid (FA) oxidation, ketone body synthesis and amino acid catabolism), apoptosis and oxidative stress pathways. SIRT3 also exists as a nuclear full length form (FL-SIRT3) that is subsequently processed to the short mitochondrial form. Therefore, SIRT3 may regulate cellular metabolism both at the transcriptional and posttranscriptional level. SIRT4 is also localized in mitochondria and acts as ADP-ribosylase. Another mitochondrial sirtuin, SIRT5, has potent demalonylation and desuccinylation enzymatic activity and is involved in the regulation of amino acid catabolism. However, the subcellular localization of SIRTs may depend on cell type and their molecular interactions, as it was shown in the case of SIRT1, SIRT2 and SIRT3, which can be found both in the nucleus and cytoplasm.

Expression of SIRTs was detected in various human tissues, including hypothalamus, liver, pancreatic islets, skeletal muscles and adipocytes. In these tissues, via modification of histones, as well as transcription factors and co-regulators, SIRTs controlled expression of other genes, particularly those involved in response to stress. It was shown that SIRTs expression and activity of SIRT enzymes are highly sensitive to several environmental factors, including CR, exercise and cold exposure, as an adaptive mechanism in response to environmental stress. Fluctuations in intracellular NAD+ levels in response to nutrient availability are believed to be a chief mediator in this phenomenon. When nutrients are plentiful, cellular metabolism relies mainly on glycolysis to produce energy, leading to generation of ATP and conversion of NAD+ to NADH. Low levels of NAD+ and high levels of NADH result in the inactivation of SIRTs enzymatic activity. In turn, CR (defined as a diet that supplies all essential nutrients, but its energetic value is reduced by 20%–40% compared with ad libitum feeding) leads to an elevation of NAD+ levels in most metabolically active tissues, resulting in increased SIRTs activity.

A growing body of literature including both in vitro and in vivo studies has implicated SIRTs in the regulation of lipid and glucose metabolism. These studies let us understand the complexity of SIRTs actions and give hope that modulation of their activity may constitute a new therapeutic strategy for the treatment of metabolic complications of obesity, such as hyperlipidemia, liver steatosis or diabetes.

SIRTs in Lipid Metabolism

SIRTs are expressed in tissues and organs involved in lipid metabolism, including liver, skeletal muscle, white (WAT) and brown (BAT) adipose tissues. In these tissues, SIRTs control lipid synthesis, storage and utilization, both directly and indirectly (via control of insulin secretion).

During fasting SIRT1 stimulates transcription of the gene encoding triglyceride lipase and subsequent lipolysis in the adipose tissue by deacetylation of peroxisome proliferator-activated receptor γ (PPARγ) co-repressors, forkhead box protein O1 (FOXO1) and PPARγ coactivator 1α (PGC1α). This process is impaired in sirt1−/− mice [12], however results of animal studies regarding sirt1 overexpression on body weight and composition are inconsistent. It is suggested that these discrepancies may be attributed to different levels of sirt1 expression between the transgenic animals as well as to differences between strains and species used in the experiments.

Fasting and cold exposure were found to increase expression of SIRT2 in WAT. That resulted in the deacetylation of FOXO1 and subsequent repression of PPARγ activity, lipolysis and the release of FA. A similar effect can be obtained by administering isoproterenol, which confirms the role of adrenergic signaling in the regulation of SIRT2 expression in WAT. SIRT2 may also inhibit lipogenesis by deacetylation of ACLY (ATP-citrate lyase), an enzyme crucial for FA synthesis. A deacetylated form of ACLY is then ubiquitinated and degraded while reducing lipogenesis.

Nutritional and thermal stress increase BAT expression of SIRT3, which regulates mitochondrial function and thermogenesis in brown adipocytes. In cultures of brown adipocyte precursors (HIB1B cells), overexpression of SIRT3 resulted in increased phosphorylation of the cAMP response element-binding protein (CREB), which then directly activated PGC-1α promoter, resulting in increased expression of the gene encoding uncoupling protein 1 (UCP1) and promotion of mitochondrial respiration. However, subsequent experiments showed that the protein produced on the basis of cDNA used in this experiment lacked proper deacetylase activity, so this finding should be treated with caution. Moreover, sirt3−/− mice, despite mitochondrial protein hyperacetylation, showed no major disturbances of adaptive thermogenesis. In contrast, livers from mice lacking sirt3 showed higher levels of FA oxidation intermediate products and triglycerides during fasting, associated with decreased levels of FA oxidation when compared with wild-type mice. These findings are consistent with the fact that deacetylation of the long-chain acyl coenzyme A dehydrogenase by SIRT3 was found to determine proper mitochondrial FA oxidation.

SIRTs in Insulin Secretion and Glucose Metabolism

SIRTs are also indirectly involved in the regulation of lipid metabolism by affecting the secretion and action of insulin, which promotes FA storage in WAT and inhibits their β-oxidation in the liver and skeletal muscle.

Insulin secretion in pancreatic β cells is related to adenosine-5′-triphosphate (ATP) production. High intracellular glucose levels result in increased synthesis of ATP, which subsequently inactivates ATP-sensitive potassium channels. The reduction of potassium efflux leads to depolarization of the plasma membrane, opening the voltage-gated calcium channels and subsequent calcium influx that stimulates insulin exocytosis. The efficiency of insulin secretion can be modulated by the uncoupling protein 2 (UCP2) that regulates intracellular levels of ATP. SIRT1 decreases expression of the gene encoding UCP2 by directly binding to its promoter. Therefore, local overexpression of sirt1 in pancreatic β cells results in enhanced insulin secretion, in response to glucose in vitro and improved glucose tolerance in vivo.

Consistently, sirt1 knock-out by RNA interference led to decreased insulin secretion in β cell lines and its systemic depletion—to impaired glucose tolerance. SIRT1, via activation of FOXO1, also participates in protecting β cells from damage-induced apoptosis. In response to toxins or to oxidative stress, FOXO1 activates expression of multiple genes to preserve insulin secretion and promote cell survival, while inhibition of SIRT1 (for example by miR-34a, whose levels increase in response to fatty acid-induced β cell dysfunction) is associated with induction of β cell apoptosis.

In contrast, SIRT4 acts as a negative regulator of insulin secretion. This mitochondrial sirtuin is selectively expressed in pancreatic β cells, were it mainly acts as a mono-ADP-ribosyltransferase. By ADP-ribosylation, SIRT4 represses the activity of glutamate dehydrogenase (GDH), an enzyme responsible for the conversion of glutamate to α-ketoglutarate, thereby promoting ATP synthesis by introducing amino acids into the tricarboxylic acid cycle. Therefore, systemic or local (for example by miR-15b) sirt4 knock-out enhances insulin secretion in response to glucose and amino acids, while its overexpression has the opposite effect. CR was found to decrease both SIRT1 and SIRT4 activity in the pancreas, not because of a decrease in their protein levels, but as a result of the decreased NAD/NADH ratio, which on the one hand reduces glucose-dependent insulin secretion and on the other hand sensitizes β cells to amino acids. This mechanism is believed to play an important role in the regulation of insulin secretion during CR that promotes deribosylation of GDH and potentates amino acid stimulated insulin secretion by β cells.

SIRTs are also involved in glycolysis and gluconeogenesis regulation. Under normal glucose availability, SIRT6 inhibits expression of multiple glycolytic genes by competing at their promoters with hypoxia induced factor 1α (HiF1α). By deacetylating histone H3 lysine 9 at promoters of Hif1α target genes, SIRT6 maintains proper glucose flux for mitochondrial respiration and prevents excessive glycolysis. In SIRT6-deficient cells, increased Hif1α activity leads to up-regulation of glycolysis and diminished mitochondrial respiration. Hepatic-specific disruption of SIRT6 by miR-33 in mice results in enhanced glycolysis and triglyceride synthesis causing liver steatosis and correlates with increased triglyceride content observed in human hepatic cell lines, transfected with miR-33. SIRT1's effect on gluconeogenesis depends on the energy resources. During short-term fasting, SIRT1 represses CRTC2 (a transcriptional coactivator for transcription factor CREB acting as a central regulator of gluconeogenic gene expression, in response to cAMP) leading to decreased gluconeogenesis. Similar effects can be obtained by interaction of SIRT1 with the signal transducer and activator of transcription 3 (STAT3) transcription factor. In contrast, when CR is prolonged, SIRT1 promotes gluconeogenesis and inhibits glycolysis by deacetylation of PGC-1α and activation of FOXO1.

SIRT1 expression may also modify insulin sensitivity; in muscle cells by transcriptional repression of the protein tyrosine phosphatase 1B gene (PTP1B, a negative regulator of the insulin signaling pathway); while in adipose tissue via an effect on glucose transporter type 4 (GLUT4) translocation, it regulates insulin-stimulated glucose uptake. Moreover, by interference with the nuclear factor κB (NF-κB) signaling pathway, SIRT1 can also repress inflammatory gene expression in adipocytes and macrophages infiltrating adipose tissue, which results in an improvement of insulin signaling pathways and a reduction of hyperinsulinemia, accompanied by increased insulin sensitivity in vivo. There is also evidence that SIRT1 may affect insulin signaling by deacetylation of the insulin receptor substrate (IRS-2) [48].

It can therefore be assumed that administration of sirtuins modulators (for example SIRT1 activators and/or SIRT4 inhibitors) can have a favorable effect on insulin secretion, while activation of SIRT6 may improve intracellular glucose metabolism and protect from insulin resistance.

CHAPTER 3 : SIRTs and Adipogenesis

Interest in SIRTs as potential targets for the treatment of obesity also results from their involvement in the regulation of adipogenesis.

PPARγ is considered a chief transcription factor responsible for promoting adipogenesis, by interacting with co-repressors of PPARγ; nuclear receptor co-repressor (N-CoR), and silencing mediator of retinoid and thyroid hormone receptors (SMRT), SIRT1 attenuates adipogenesis. Consistently, overexpression of ectopic sirt1 blocks adipogenesis in 3T3-L1 cells, a culture of mouse adipocytes was used as a model of adipocyte differentiation. Additionally, via activation of the Wnt signaling pathway, SIRT1 determinates mesenchymal stem cell (MSC) differentiation towards myogenic cells, while its inhibition in MSC promotes adipogenesis.

One concept of obesity treatment is based on the activation of preadipocyte genes specific to BAT, which is characterized by high metabolic activity. Since SIRT1, by direct deacetylation of PPARγ, recruits the BAT program coactivator Prdm16 to PPARγ, it also plays a crucial role in the induction of genes typical for BAT and repression of visceral WAT genes associated with insulin resistance. Therefore, silencing of sirt1 in 3T3-L1 preadipocytes leads to their hyperplasia and increased expression of WAT and inflammatory markers with a parallel decrease in BAT markers. Recent studies underlined the role of different miRNAs as negative regulators of SIRT1 during adipocyte differentiation, for example miR-34a, miR-146b, miR-181a, suggesting that interference with these miRNAs may constitute a therapeutic approach in the treatment of excess adiposity, as well as in the activation of brown adipocytes .

Another sirtuin family member, SIRT2, was also shown to exert an inhibitory effect on adipocyte differentiation. This process is mediated by FOXO1 deacetylation and subsequent PPARγ transcriptional activity repression. Therefore, sirt2 overexpression inhibits adipogenesis, while its silencing has an opposite effect in 3T3-L1 preadipocytes. This inhibitory effect of SIRT2 on adipocyte differentiation discloses under nutritional stress suggesting that combination of SIRT2 activators with diet could provide novel therapeutic strategy for obesity.

In vitro studies showed that SIRT7 is required for PPARγ expression and proper adipocyte differentiation. Unlike SIRT1 and SIRT2, its deletion or downregulation diminishes the ability of mouse embryo fibroblasts and 3T3L1 cells to undergo adipogenesis. However, its overexpression did not restore preadipocyte differentiation, suggesting that SIRT7 is required but not sufficient to perform a full program of adipogenesis. Interestingly, SIRT7 is a metabolic target for miR-93, a negative regulator of adipogenesis, whose expression is decreased in genetically obese ob/ob mice. This miRNA was also found to be a key regulator of mature adipocyte turnover and its inhibition increases fat tissue formation in vivo.

Therefore, it can be expected that in the future activation of SIRT1 and SIRT2 or inhibition of SIRT7 by appropriate miRNA, may be a therapeutic strategy for the treatment of obesity.

Animal Studies

As described above, in vitro studies have shown the important role of SIRT enzymes in the regulation of glucose and lipid metabolism as well as in the control of adipogenesis. In vivo studies, in which particular genes encoding SIRTs were either silenced or overexpressed in experimental animals, have provided further data on the role of SIRTs in the pathogenesis of obesity. Additionally, abnormalities of SIRTs' action were also investigated in different animal models of obesity.

SIRT1 deficiency may result in different phenotypes. Complete, systemic knock-out of sirt1 in inbred mice leads to serious developmental defects, sterility and high postnatal lethality; whereby these animals are not appropriate for the study of energy metabolism. However, some of the outbred sirt1−/− mice reached adulthood and due to the hypermetabolic state have significantly lower body weight compared to wild-type animals [56]. The heterozygous sirt1+/− mice develop and reproduce normally, and when fed a high-fat diet have increased body and liver fat content, reduced energy expenditure, elevated inflammatory parameters in sera, adipose tissue and liver that resemble the metabolic syndrome phenotype.

Liver-specific sirt1 knock-down in mice on CR results in lower systemic cholesterol levels and increased liver accumulation of cholesterol and FA. However, results regarding the metabolic consequences of a high-calorie diet in these animals are contradictory. While some researchers reported that they have lower liver steatosis rates than wild-type controls bred in the same manner, others claim that liver-specific sirt1 knock-down in mice is associated with severe liver steatosis and inflammatory infiltrations .

Specific genetic ablation of sirt1 in WAT leads to obesity, increased inflammatory infiltration, and insulin resistance similar to that observed in high-fat diet induced obesity. However, in a recent study, adipocyte-specific knock-out of sirt1 in short-term observation led to an exacerbation of metabolic complications, while it improved metabolic functions long-term. The authors of the study suggested that this phenomenon is related to the obesity-associated unphosporylation of PPARγ that induces a set of target genes which can promote insulin sensitivity.

In contrast, transgenic mice moderately overexpressing sirt1 under the control of a β-actin promoter develop a phenotype similar to mice on CR. They gain less body weight and have reduced levels of serum cholesterol, glucose and insulin compared with littermate controls, and are protected against the negative metabolic consequences of a high-fat diet. However, when sirt1 is overexpressed under its own promoter, the animals, despite decreased food intake, have normal body weight due to lower energy expenditure and are not protected from diet-induced obesity.

Although a detailed presentation of studies on the role of SIRTs in the central regulation of appetite is beyond the scope of this paper, it should be mentioned that while animal studies suggest that peripheral actions of SIRT1 mostly promote a negative energy balance, its role in the central regulation of metabolism is less clear. On the one hand, CR leads to increased expression of sirt1 in hypothalamic nuclei in mice, especially in the arcuate nucleus (ARC) producing anorexigenic proopiomelanocortin (POMC) and orexigenic peptides, including neuropeptide Y (NPY) and aguit-related peptide (AgRP). Consistently, targeted sirt1 overexpression in the hypothalamus results in a similar phenotype and biochemical profile as in animals on a hypocaloric diet . Overexpression of sirt1 in mouse POMC or AgRP neurons also prevents age-associated weight gain in two different manners: in POMC neurons it stimulates energy expenditure via increased sympathetic activity in adipose tissue and in AgRP neurons, it suppresses food intake. These beneficial results are diminished in aging mice and mice consuming an high-fat, high-sucrose diet due to decreases in SIRT1 and NAD+ levels in the hypothalamus. This shows that age and obesity-related decline in ARC SIRT1 function contributes to a disruption of energy homeostasis .

On the other hand, there are studies that suggest that in the central neural system SIRT1 promotes a positive energy balance. Mice with neuron-specific sirt1 knock-out (SINKO) are protected against the metabolic complications of a high-fat diet that include lower fasting insulin levels, improved glucose tolerance, enhanced systemic and central insulin sensitivity compared with wild-type animals, suggesting that neuronal SIRT1 negatively regulates hypothalamic insulin signaling, leading to systemic insulin resistance. Consistently, acute inhibition of SIRT1 by intracerebroventricular injection of its inhibitor (Ex-527) in rodents results in long-term reduced food intake and body weight gain, which is accompanied by an increase in POMC levels and a decrease in AgRP in ARC . These findings are contributed to a SIRT1-mediated reduction of FOXO-1 activity that positively regulates transcription of genes encoding AgRP and NPY and decreases expression of POMC. Collectively, these results suggest that in the hypothalamus SIRT1, via its effect on FOXO1, may promote cell-specific functions that result in divergent adaptive, metabolic responses. Taking the above data into account, even though approaches aimed at enhancing peripheral SIRT1 activity while reducing its central action, may seem attractive in the treatment of obesity, their use in clinical practice requires more detailed knowledge of the SIRT1 function in distinct organs and tissues.

Compared with SIRT1, knowledge about the role of other SIRTs in the pathogenesis of obesity is relatively limited. Nevertheless, recent years have brought new data from animal models suggesting that SIRT2-7 are also important in this aspect.

Human Studies

The knowledge of the role of SIRTs in the regulation of metabolism comes primarily from animal studies. The number of publications on the role of SIRTs in regulating metabolism in humans is limited and can be classified into two categories: studies on SIRTs expression in metabolically active tissues and genetic studies concerning the association between polymorphisms in SIRTs and development of obesity in humans.

Human Obesity Associated Changes in SIRTs Expression

Human studies suggest that obesity is accompanied by alternations of SIRTs levels in distinct tissues and organs.

Transcript levels of SIRT1 in adipose tissue and peripheral blood mononuclear cells (PBMC) are significantly lower in obese individuals, compared with normal-weight controls that can be successfully restored by weight loss obtained either by CR or bariatric surgery. Since SIRT1 increases lipolysis and suppresses inflammatory responses, it is plausible that its decreased expression in the adipose tissue of obese individuals might be associated with excessive fat accumulation and development of obesity-related inflammation. This hypothesis is supported by the fact that the lowest SIRT1 mRNA levels can be found in adipose tissues from obese patients diagnosed with T2DM and severe hepatic steatosis.

Weight loss is also associated with increased SIRT3 and SIRT6 mRNA levels in liver and subcutaneous adipose tissues of morbidly obese individuals. This finding is consistent with the abovementioned animal studies, where diet-induced fatty liver disease is accompanied by reduced SIRT3 activity. While mice overexpressing sirt6, despite a high-fat diet, accumulate less visceral fat, have a more favorable lipid profile and enhanced glucose tolerance compared with wild-type controls.

SIRT4 mRNA levels in serum and PBMC are inversely correlated with different anthropometric parameters (BMI, waist circumference, fat mass) as well as with insulin, cholesterol and triglyceride concentrations. However, simultaneous analysis of the growth hormone/IGF-1 axis revealed that these relations are probably secondary to the low GH and IGF-1 levels observed in obese individuals, both involved in the regulation of SIRT4 status. Nevertheless, according to the hypothesis that mitochondrial functions are adjusted to environmental requirements, it is suggested that low serum SIRT4 levels in obesity occur in response to calorie excess in order to decrease fat oxidative capacity in the liver and muscles, but promote excess ectopic lipid storage.

In contrast, mean mRNA levels of SIRT7 are higher in adipose tissues obtained from obese individuals than in those of normal-weight controls Knowledge about the role of SIRT7 in the pathogenesis of human obesity is still unclear and its expression in human adipose tissue has not been previously documented. As mentioned above, in rodents sirt7 knock-out led to resistance to high-fat diet-induced obesity, liver steatosis and glucose intolerance; however these abnormalities may result from impaired PPARγ expression. Some data also suggests an interaction between SIRT1 and SIRT7 at the molecular level, as was shown in immunoprecipitation assays and in vivo, where SIRT1 protein levels and enzymatic activity were increased in WAT of animals with sirt7 knock-out. In our work, we also observed a negative correlation between SIRT1 and SIRT7 mRNA levels in adipose tissues from obese individuals. Since it is suggested that SIRT7 inhibits SIRT1 auto-deacetylation and restricts its activity, the proper balance between these two sirtuins may be therefore crucial for the maintenance of metabolic homeostasis.

Although there is growing evidence pointing to the role of SIRTs in the regulation of different metabolic pathways in humans, the factors that control their expression in adipose tissues are less known. In our research, we detected a negative correlation between SIRT1 and SIRT7 mRNA levels and the levels of relevant miRNAs, the role of which in the regulation of expression of these genes had been previously demonstrated in vitro. With respect to SIRT1, we observed that its lower expression in adipose tissues of obese individuals correlated negatively with levels of miR-34a (which is physiologically up-regulated in mature adipocytes), and with two miRNA that have opposite effect on adipocyte differentiation: miR-22 (inhibiting adipogenic differentiation by targeting histone deacetylase 6) and miR-181a (promoting adipocyte differentiation by inhibition of the tumor necrosis factor α pathway). In turn, in our study, SIRT7 targeting miR-125a was under-expressed in obese individuals and this finding was consistent with animal studies where down-regulation of this miRNA in murine adipocytes was associated with insulin resistance. In contrast, we found no association between CpG methylation status of the SIRT1 and SIRT7 regulatory regions and their expression on the mRNA level in adipose tissues, so it is possible that methylation does not play a crucial role in obesity-associated changes in SIRTs expression in humans .

Given their role in the regulation of lipid and glucose metabolism, adipogenesis and appetite control SIRTs constitute promising targets for novel therapies of obesity and associated metabolic disorders. However, the discovery of a single compound that would be able to activate some SIRTs isoforms and inhibit others is still a challenge. Another difficulty is to obtain tissue action specificity for these compounds, since SIRTs activity may depend on cell type and environmental factors.

Possible applications of SIRTs' inhibitors include, among others, treatment of cancer, immunodeficiency virus infection or neurodegenerative disorders. Until now, the only aspects in which SIRTs inhibitors could be used to treat obesity-associated metabolic disorders was inducing favorable changes in body composition. SIRT1 inhibiting compounds, such as splitomycin, suramin, salermide, EX-527 or sirtinol, can be used to increase the amount of skeletal muscle. This concept is based on animal studies where sirt1−/− mice display higher muscle growth compared with wild-type animals and mice with muscle specific sirt1 overexpression. However, SIRT1 inhibitors have not been tested for that purpose in humans.

The first invented compound that was able to activate SIRT1 in a way that mimics CR was the polyphenol Resveratrol (RSV). In vitro studies demonstrated that RSV is able to successfully inhibit preadipocyte maturation and induce adipocyte apoptosis. However, the pro-apoptotic proprieties of RSV were observed predominantly in concentrations that may be difficult to obtain with its systemic administration in vivo. Therefore, this effect of RSV on adipose tissue can be difficult to apply in clinical practice. The potential anti-obesity effects of RSV may also result from its influence on lipid metabolism in the liver and skeletal muscle. In skeletal muscle, by activation of PGC-1α, RSV stimulates mitochondrial activity, including β-oxidation of FA. Its administration to rodents on high fat diet protects from intramuscular lipid accumulation and insulin resistance. Similarly in the liver, by activation of the AMPK-SIRT1 axis leading to increased β-oxidation of FA and to decreased lipogenesis, RSV prevents rodents from steatosis induced by a high fat or high calorie diet. A composition containing RSV, leucine, β-hydroxymethylbutrate (HMB) and keto-isocaproic acid, has been recently patented to synergistically activate SIRT1 and SIRT3 in order to induce FA oxidation and mitochondrial biogenesis. This combination when tested on 3LT3-L1 preadipocytes was more effective in the activation of SIRT1 than RSV alone, but was also able to activate SIRT3. In c57/BL6 mice, treatment with a combination of low doses of RSV with either HMB or leucine resulted in reduction of body weight and improvement of body composition accompanied by increased insulin sensitivity. In turn, a combination of RSV with HMB and metformin was highly effective in increasing myotube FA oxidation. Summarizing, in rodents RSV has proved to be effective in the reduction of adipose tissue content by inhibiting the fat accumulation processes and stimulating the lipolytic pathways. Nevertheless, it is still being investigated whether the results of in vivo studies can be extrapolated to humans.

A reformulated version of RSV, with improved bioavailability, when administered to 11 obese men for 30 days exerted several favorable metabolic effects similar to those that can be obtained by CR or increased physical activity. These changes included a reduction of blood pressure, hepatic lipid content as well as serum glucose, triglyceride and inflammatory marker levels with a parallel improvement in skeletal muscle mitochondrial function. RSV treatment also changed the subcutaneous adipose tissue morphology and function. It increased the number of small adipocytes and caused up-regulation of genes involved in lipid breakdown by autophagy . What is important, the compound was well tolerated at the tested concentration and no adverse events were reported.

Another micronized formulation of RSV, SRT501, via activation of the similar set of genes as in the case of CR, was able to counteract the negative consequences of a high calorie diet in mice as well as lower glucose levels and increase insulin sensitivity in patients with T2DM. This effect of RSV was confirmed by a recent study where its 12 week-long administration to 10 subjects with T2DM resulted in an increase of SIRT1 and AMPK expression in muscles accompanied by an increase of the basic metabolic rate. The same treatment in patients with non-alcoholic fatty liver disease reduced the alanine transaminase level and hepatic steatosis but had no beneficial effect on anthropometric parameters, markers of insulin resistance, lipid profile or blood pressure.

However, there are also clinical trials that question the effectiveness of RSV in obesity treatment. In a randomized, placebo-controlled, double-blinded study on 24 obese but otherwise healthy men, 4-week-long administration of RSV had no significant effect on insulin sensitivity, blood pressure, basic metabolic rate, body composition or inflammatory parameters. While administration of RSV in the treatment of obesity can be considered an encouraging therapeutic approach, its prophylactic administration to individuals with normal BMI does not seem to be founded. Twelve-week-long RSV supplementation to non-obese, postmenopausal women with normal glucose tolerance did not affect body composition, basic metabolic rate or plasma levels of metabolic and inflammatory markers. Major limitations of the abovementioned studies are the small numbers of participants and relatively short follow-up time; therefore, further studies to investigate the long-term and dose-dependent metabolic effects of RSV supplementation on larger cohorts are needed.

Compounds other than resveratrol also proved their effectiveness in activating SIRT1. One example is SRT2104, a compound with anti-inflammatory properties that improves glucose homeostasis and increases insulin sensitivity in animal models; however, its administration to patients with T2DM did not lead to any consistent, dose-related changes in glucose or insulin levels. Another example of small molecule activators of SIRT1 is SRT1720, which is able to increase deacetylation of SIRT1 substrates in vitro and was successfully applied in vivo to treat insulin resistance in several animal models of type 2 diabetes: diet induced obesity (DIO) mice, genetically obese ob/ob mice, and Zucker fa/fa rats in a concentration 10-fold lower than SRT501. Apart from a favorable effect on glucose metabolism, by decreasing lipogenic gene expression, SRT1720 was effective in the treatment of animal models of liver steatosis. However, there are also studies that question the beneficial effect of SRT1720 on metabolic parameters in animals fed a high-fat diet. Moreover, in biochemical assays with native substrates and in biophysical studies, RSV and other SIRT1 activators (SRT1720, SRT2183, SRT1460) were found not to activate SIRT1 directly. It is postulated that indirect activation of RSV is mediated by the activation of AMPK, which increases intracellular NAD+ levels and thus induces deacetylation of SIRT1 targets. However, there is also data demonstrating the direct interaction of RSV derivates with the SIRT1 enzyme molecule, since SIRT1 mutations can significantly reduce their activity. Apart from the controversy regarding the mechanism of their action, another issue that may raise concerns with the use of RSV derivates in everyday practice is their target promiscuity that may result in unexpected adverse effects. As a result, SIRTs modulators are still under consideration before they can be approved for routine treatment of obesity and metabolic disorders.

The more is known about the effects of SIRTs on energy balance, lipid and glucose metabolism, adipogenesis regulation as well as their impaired activity in animal and human obesity, the more attractive is the idea that their activators and inhibitors may be useful in the treatment of obesity and associated complications. Data from transgenic animal studies that proved that there are benefits derived from the activation of particular SIRT enzymes is especially encouraging. However, one should remember that SIRTs' activities are not limited to the metabolism regulation and include, among others, control of longevity, oncogenesis as well as neurological and cardiovascular functions.

PART TWO: THE SIRTFOOD DIET
CHAPTER 6: What Is The SIRTfood Diet?

The Sirtfood Diet was created by nutritionists Aiden Goggins and Glen Matten. They were so interested by the potential of Sirtfoods, they created a diet based around maximising Sirtfood intake and mild calorie restriction. They then tested this diet on participants from an exclusive London gym and were amazed by their findings. Gym members lost an average of 7lbs in the first 7 days, despite not increasing their levels of exercise. Not only did the participants lose a substantial amount of weight, but they also gained muscle (usually the opposite happens when dieting) and reported significant improvements in overall health and well-being.

The Sirtfood diet is really not just another new trendy or fad diet. The principle of the diet is to bring about the knowledge of foods and how the health impact the nutrients you take in can be of benefit to your body. As Sirtfoods are natural they can be incorporated into your current diet – whether you favor a whole foods diet, paleo or another diet – there's no disputing that these foods have remarkable health benefits.

Although the early stage of juicing and fasting seems just good for those who might want to lose a little weight quickly, the general aim of the Sirtfood diet is to include healthier foods into your diet to increase your well being and boost your immune system.

So while the first seven days seem very difficult, the longer-term plan can work for everyone.

By focusing on introducing Sirtfood- rich ingredients into your everyday meals you can continue the fat burning whilst enjoying your regular favorites.

All this raises the question: What can we do to activate sirtuins and reap these amazing benefits? It is well-known that both fasting and exercise activate sirtuins. But alas, both demand an unwavering commitment to either food restriction or demanding exercise regimes. Cutting back on calories leaves us feeling fatigued, hungry, and decidedly cranky, and in the longer term can lead to muscle loss and a stagnant metabolism. As for exercise, the amount needed to be effective for weight loss requires a LOT of effort. Both can be hard to accomplish.

In 2013, the results of one of the most prestigious nutritional studies ever carried out were published. The premise of the study, called PREDIMED, was beautifully simple: It studied the difference between a Mediterranean-style diet supplemented with either extra-virgin olive oil or nuts and a more conventional modern diet. Results showed that after five years, heart disease and diabetes were slashed by an incredible 30 percent, along with major reductions in the risk of obesity in the Mediterranean diet group. This wasn't surprising, but when the study was investigated in greater detail it was discovered there was no difference in calorie, fat, or carbohydrate intake between the two groups. How do you explain that?

Not all (healthy) foods are created equal.

Research now shows that plants contain natural compounds called polyphenols that have immense benefits for our health. And when researchers analyzing PREDIMED investigated polyphenol consumption among the participants, the results were staggering. Over just the five-year period, those who consumed the highest levels of polyphenols had 37 percent fewer deaths compared to those who ate the least.

But not all polyphenols are equal. Data out of Harvard University from over 124,000 individuals showed that only certain polyphenols were helpful for weight control. Similarly, a study of almost 3,000 twins found that a higher intake of only certain polyphenols was linked with less body fat and a healthier distribution of fat in the body. Polyphenols are undoubtedly a boon for staying slim and healthy, but if not all polyphenols are equal, then which are the best? Could it be those that research has shown have the ability to switch on our sirtuin genes? The very same ones activated by fasting and exercise?

The pharmaceutical industry has been quick to exploit these sirtuin-activating nutrients, investing hundreds of millions to convert them into panacea drugs. For example, the popular diabetes drug metformin comes from a plant and activates our sirtuin genes. But until now they have been largely overlooked by the world of nutrition, to the detriment of our health and our waistlines.

CHAPTER 8: What Foods Activate Sirtuins?

With our interest piqued we put all the foods with the highest levels of sirtuin-activating polyphenols together into a special diet. This includes extra-virgin olive oil and walnuts, the specific inclusions in PREDIMED, as well as arugula, red onions, strawberries, red wine, dark chocolate, green tea, and coffee among many others. When we pilot tested it, the results were stunning. Participants lost weight, while either maintaining or even increasing their muscle mass. Best of all, people reported feeling great—brimming with energy, sleeping better, and with notable improvements in their skin.

And so the Sirtfood Diet was born, a revolutionary new way to activate sirtuins by eating delicious foods. A diet that doesn't involve calorie counting, cutting out carbs, or eating low fat. A diet of inclusion in which you reap the benefits from eating the foods your love. The Sirtfood Diet is challenging the status quo of healthy eating advice and what it really means to look and feel great. And all from eating our favorite foods!

CHAPTER 9: The Top 20 Sirtfoods

Lots of foods contain sirtuin-activating nutrients, but some contain more than others. In this book 'The Sirtfood Diet', the authors of the diet list the 20 best Sirtfoods, these are: birds-eye chillies, buckwheat, capers, celery, cocoa, coffee, extra virgin olive oil, green tea, kale, lovage, medjool dates, parsley, red chicory, red wine, rocket, soy, strawberries, turmeric and walnuts.

CHAPTER 10: How Does The SIRTfood Diet Work?

The diet is split into 2 phases. Phase 1: the 7 day 'hypersuccess phase', which combines a Sirtfood-rich diet with moderate calorie restriction, and Phase 2: the 14 day 'maintenance phase', where you consolidate your weight loss without restricting calories.

PHASE 1 OF THE SIRTFOOD DIET

During the first 3 days, calorie intake is restricted to 1,000 calories (so, still more than on a 5:2 fasting day). The diet consists of 3 Sirtfood-rich green juices and 1 Sirtfood-rich meal and 2 squares of dark chocolate.

During the remaining 4 days, calorie intake is increased to 1, 500 calories and each day the diet comprises 2 Sirtfood-rich green juices and 2 Sirtfood-rich meals.

During phase 1 you are not allowed to drink any alcohol, but you can drink water, tea, coffee and green tea freely.

PHASE 2 OF THE SIRTFOOD DIET

Phase 2 does not focus on calorie restriction. Each day involves 3 Sirtfood-rich meals and 1 green juice, plus the option of 1 or 2 Sirtfood bite snacks, if required.

In phase 2 you are allowed to drink red wine, but in moderation (the recommendation is 2-3 glasses of red wine per week), as well as water, tea, coffee and green tea.

You may repeat the two phases as often as you would like to meet your weight loss goals. Even if you have achieved it, the creators of the diet suggest adopting sirtfoods for your day-to-day needs because they have designed this diet as an alternative way of living.

This means that after the first three weeks, you are encouraged to keep having meals and green juices that are rich in sirtfoods. Other than this, here are some more things that you can do to get more and continue reaping the benefits of sirtfoods for your health:

- Resume your workout routines.

Since your calorie limit for the first couple of weeks into the diet, it is best to either lessen or stop working out while your body gets used to its new condition. No two persons are exactly alike, so the best thing you can do to know when you can start exercising like you usually do it by paying closer attention to your body.

To be on the safer side of things, most followers opt to resume their regular workout schedule after clearing phase 2 of the diet. By then, you would feel more energized, and more capable of completing your usual exercise sets.

Take note that even though a sirtfood diet does not require you to exercise to unlock its benefits, it would still be best for the overall wellness of your body and mind to remain fit and active every day.

- Try out sirtfood smoothies with protein powder.

If you decide to start exercising again, you should add smoothies that contain lots of sirtfoods and protein powder to help you reduce the soreness of your muscles, and keep you well energized throughout and after your workout.

Recipes for fun and tasty sirtfood smoothies can easily be found in blogs and recipe books dedicated to the Sirtfood Diet. If you are pretty confident with your skills in the kitchen, then feel free to experiment with the recommended ingredients, and discover the perfect smoothie combinations for your taste buds.

- Invite your family and friends to try out the diet.

One of the best ways to maintain your healthier diet is by getting the people around you involved in it as well. Studies show that the kind of company you keep can have a huge influence on your lifestyle, including what and how you eat.

Ideally, you can try convincing them by showing the positive effects that the Sirtfood Diet has had on you. Let them also read this guide so that they will have a better idea of what it is, what it can do for them, and how they should go about it.

Consider adopting the principles of the Sirtfood Diet as part of your way of life. It is just not a one-time, quick-fix meal plan, and you cannot go wrong by adding more sirtfoods into your day-to-day diet.

Is it healthy and sustainable?

Sirtfoods are nearly all healthy options and may even lead to some health benefits due to their anti-inflammatory or antioxidant residential or commercial properties.

The Sirtfood Diet is needlessly restrictive and uses no clear, special health benefits over any other kind of diet.

Eating only 1,000 calories is normally not suggested without the supervision of a physician. Even consuming 1,500 calories per day is exceedingly limiting for many individuals.

The diet plan also needs draining to 3 green juices per day. Although juices can be a good source of minerals and vitamins, they are likewise a source of sugar and consist of nearly none of the healthy fiber that whole fruits and veggies do

What's more, sipping on juice throughout the whole day is a bad concept for both your blood sugar and your teeth.

Not to point out, because the diet plan is so minimal in calories and food choice, it is more than most likely lacking in protein, vitamins and minerals, specifically during the first stage.

Due to the low calorie levels and limiting food options, this diet plan may be challenging to adhere to for the whole three weeks.

Add that to the high initial expenses of needing to buy a juicer, the book and specific uncommon and costly components, and this diet plan ends up being unfeasible and unsustainable for many individuals.

The Sirtfood Diet promotes healthy foods but is limiting in calories and food choices. It likewise involves drinking great deals of juice, which isn't a healthy suggestion.

Joining Exercise with The Sirtfood Diet

With 52% of Americans admitting that they think that its simpler to do their charges than to see how to eat steadily, it's fundamental to present a type of eating that turns into a lifestyle as opposed to a coincidental prevailing fashion diet. For a few of us it may not be that difficult to get thinner or hold a solid weight, however the Sirtfood diet can help the individuals who are battling. Be that as it may, shouldn't something be said about joining the Sirtfood diet with work out, is it fitting to stay away from practice totally or present it once you have begun the diet?

The SirtDiet Principles

With an expected 650 million hefty grown-ups internationally, it's critical to discover smart dieting and exercise systems that are feasible, don't deny you of all that you appreciate, and don't expect you to practice all week. The Sirtfood diet does only that. The thought is that sure nourishments will dynamic the 'thin quality' pathways which are normally actuated by fasting and exercise. Fortunately certain nourishment and drink, including dull chocolate and red wine, contain synthetic substances called polyphenols that enact the qualities that copy the impacts of activity and fasting.

Exercise during the initial barely any weeks

During the main week or two of the diet where your calorie admission is diminished, it is reasonable to stop or lessen practice while your body adjusts to less calories. Tune in to your body and if you feel exhausted or have less vitality than expected, don't work out. Rather guarantee that you stay concentrated on the rules that apply to a solid lifestyle, for example, including satisfactory day by day levels of fiber, protein and products of the soil.

When the diet turns into a lifestyle

When you do practice it's critical to devour protein in a perfect world an hour after your workout. Protein fixes muscles after exercise, lessens irritation and can help recuperation. There are an assortment of plans which incorporate protein which will be ideal for post-practice utilization, for example, the sirt stew con carne or the turmeric chicken and kale serving of mixed greens. If you need something lighter you could attempt the sirt blueberry smoothie and include some protein powder for included advantage. The kind of wellness you do will be down to you, however workouts at home will permit you to pick when to work out, the sorts of activities that suit you and are short and helpful.

The Sirtfood diet is incredible approach to change your dietary patterns, shed pounds and feel more advantageous. The underlying not many weeks may challenge you yet it's imperative to check which nourishments are ideal to eat and which scrumptious plans suit you. Be benevolent to yourself in the initial barely any weeks while your body adjusts and take practice simple if you decide to do it by any stretch of the imagination. If you are as of now somebody who moderates or extreme exercise then it might be that you can carry on as ordinary, or deal with your wellness as per the adjustment in diet. Similarly as with any diet and exercise changes, it's about the individual and how far you can propel yourself.

Minerals and nutrients for which ladies may require supplements incorporate calcium, iron, Vitamins B6, B12 and D. Men, be that as it may, need to focus on fiber, magnesium, Vitamins B9, C and E.

That reason applies to weight loss diets also. People's nourishment necessities sway which weight loss diets are increasingly compelling for each sex.

If you're similar to the vast majority, you've seen an astounding number of weight loss projects and patterns go back and forth; practically every one of them have their benefits and practically every one of them work — incidentally. Weight the executives and therapeutic experts fight collectively that the deep rooted, proven blend of good sustenance and ordinary exercise is the most ideal approach to adequately shed pounds and keep it off.

The Sirtfood Diet is not designed to be a one off 'diet' but rather a way of life. You are encouraged, once you've completed the first 3 weeks, to continue eating a diet rich in Sirtfoods and to continue drinking your daily green juice. This Sirtfood Diet Book, with recipes for lots more Sirtfood-rich main meals, as well as recipes for alternatives to the green juice and more hints and tips for following the Sirtfood Diet. There are even some recipes for Sirtfood desserts! The authors of The Sirtfood Diet suggest that Phases 1 and 2 can be repeated as and when necessary for a health boost, or if things have gone a bit off track.

CHAPTER 11: The 7-DAY MEAL PLAN

You can do this plan for up to two weeks, after which it's all about adjusting it to suit your lifestyle.There are no set rules – just try to include as many sirtfoods as possible in your diet, which should make you feel healthier, more energetic and improve your skin, as well as making you leaner.

This super-healthy green juice and these yummy choc balls are Sirtfood Diet staples.

All recipes serve one (unless otherwise stated).

Sirtfood Green Juice

Ingredients:

- 75g kale
- 30g rocket
- 5g flat-leaf parsley
- 5g lovage leaves (optional)
- 150g celery, including leaves
- 1/2 medium green apple
- Juice 1/2 lemon
- 1/2tsp matcha green tea

Directions:

1. Juice the kale, rocket, parsley and lovage, if using, then add the celery and apple and blend again. Squeeze in the lemon.
2. Pour a small amount of the juice into a glass, then add the matcha and stir until dissolved. Add the remaining juice and serve immediately.

NOTE: Only use matcha in the first two drinks of the day, as it contains the same caffeine content as a normal cup of tea. If you're not used to it, it may keep you awake if drunk later in the day.

Sirtfood Bites (makes 15-20 bites)

Ingredients:

- 120g walnuts
- 30g dark chocolate (85% cocoa solids), broken into pieces, or cocoa nibs
- 250g Medjool dates, pitted
- 1tbsp cocoa powder
- 1tbsp ground turmeric
- 1tbsp extra virgin olive oil
- Scraped seeds of 1 vanilla pod or 1tsp vanilla extract

Directions:

1. Place the walnuts and chocolate into a food processor and blend until you have a fine powder. Add all the other ingredients and blend until the mixture forms a large ball. Add 2tbsp water to help bind it, if needed.
2. Using your hands, make bite-sized balls from the mix and refrigerate in an airtight container for at least 1 hour before serving. The balls will keep for up to a week in the fridge.

Day 1

3 x sirtfood green juices

2 x sirtfood bites (you can substitute these for 15-20g of dark chocolate if you wish)

1 x sirtfood meal

Asian king prawn stir-fry

Ingredients:

- 150g raw king prawns, shelled
- 2tsp tamari or soy sauce
- 2tsp extra virgin olive oil
- 1 clove garlic, finely chopped
- 1 bird's eye chilli, finely chopped
- 1tsp fresh ginger, finely chopped
- 20g red onion, sliced
- 40g celery, trimmed and sliced
- 75g green beans, chopped
- 50g kale, roughly chopped
- 100ml chicken stock
- 75g soba (buckwheat noodles)
- 5g lovage or celery leaves

Directions:

1. In a frying pan over a high heat, cook the prawns in 1tsp tamari or soy sauce and 1tsp oil for 2-3 minutes. Transfer to a plate.
2. Add the remaining oil to the pan and fry the garlic, chilli, ginger, red onion, celery, beans and kale over a medium-high heat for 2-3 minutes. Add the stock and bring to the boil, then simmer until the vegetables are cooked but still crunchy.
3. Cook the noodles in boiling water according to pack instructions. Drain and add the lovage or celery leaves, noodles and prawns to the pan. Bring back to the boil, then remove from the heat and serve.

Day 2

3 x sirtfood green juices   2 x sirtfood bites   1 x sirtfood meal

Turkey escalope

Ingredients:

- 150g cauliflower, roughly chopped
- 1 clove garlic, finely chopped
- 40g red onion, finely chopped
- 1 bird's eye chilli, finely chopped
- 1tsp fresh ginger, finely chopped
- 2tbsp extra virgin olive oil
- 2tsp ground turmeric
- 30g sun-dried tomatoes, finely chopped
- 10g parsley
- 150g turkey escalope
- 1tsp dried sage
- Juice 1/2 lemon
- 1tbsp capers

Directions:

1. Place the cauliflower in a food processor and pulse in 2-second bursts to finely chop it until it resembles couscous. Set aside. Fry the garlic, red onion, chilli and ginger in 1tsp of the oil until soft but not coloured. Add the turmeric and cauliflower and cook for 1 minute. Remove from the heat and add the sun-dried tomatoes and half the parsley.
2. Coat the turkey escalope in the remaining oil and sage then fry for 5-6 minutes, turning regularly. When cooked, add the lemon juice, remaining parsley, capers and 1tbsp water to the pan to make a sauce, then serve.

Day 3

3 x sirtfood green juices   2 x sirtfood bites   1 x sirtfood meal

Aromatic chicken

Ingredients:

For the salsa

- 1 large tomato
- 1 bird's eye chilli, finely chopped
- 1tbsp capers, finely chopped
- 5g parsley, finely chopped
- Juice 1/2 lemon

For the chicken

- 120g skinless, boneless chicken breast
- 2tsp ground turmeric
- Juice 1/2 lemon
- 1tbsp extra virgin olive oil
- 50g kale, chopped
- 20g red onion, sliced
- 1tsp fresh ginger, finely chopped
- 50g buckwheat

Directions:

1. Heat the oven to 220ºC/200ºC fan/gas mark 7.
2. To make the salsa, finely chop the tomato, making sure you keep as much of the liquid as possible. Mix with the chilli, capers, parsley and lemon juice.
3. Marinate the chicken breast in 1tsp of the turmeric, lemon juice and half the oil for 5-10 minutes.
4. Heat an ovenproof frying pan, add the marinated chicken and cook for a minute on each side until golden, then transfer to the oven for 8-10 minutes or until cooked through. Remove, cover with foil and leave to rest for 5 minutes.
5. Cook the kale in a steamer for 5 minutes. Fry the onion and ginger in the rest of the oil until soft but not coloured, then add the cooked kale and fry for another minute.
6. Cook the buckwheat according to pack instructions with the remaining turmeric, and serve.

Day 4

2 x sirtfood green juices   2 x sirtfood meals

Sirt Muesli

Ingredients:

- 20g buckwheat flakes
- 10g buckwheat puffs
- 15g coconut flakes or desiccated coconut
- 40g Medjool dates, pitted and chopped
- 15g walnuts, chopped
- 10g cocoa nibs
- 100g strawberries, hulled and chopped
- 100g plain Greek yoghurt (or vegan alternative, such as soya or coconut yoghurt)

Directions:

1. Mix all of the ingredients together and serve (leaving out the strawberries and yoghurt if not serving straight away).

Pan-fried salmon salad

Ingredients:

For the dressing

- 10g parsley
- Juice 1/2 lemon
- 1tbsp capers
- 1tbsp extra virgin olive oil

For the salad

- 1/2 avocado, peeled, stoned and diced
- 100g cherry tomatoes, halved
- 20g red onion, thinly sliced
- 50g rocket
- 5g celery leaves

- 150g skinless salmon fillet
- 2tsp brown sugar
- 70g chicory (head), halved lengthways

Directions:

1. Heat the oven to 220ºC/ 200ºC fan/gas mark 7.
2. To make the dressing, whizz the parsley, lemon juice, capers and 2tsp oil in a blender until smooth.
3. For the salad, mix the avocado, tomato, red onion, rocket and celery leaves together.
4. Rub the salmon with a little oil and sear it in an ovenproof frying pan for a minute. Transfer to a baking tray and cook in the oven for 5 minutes.
5. Mix the brown sugar with 1tsp oil and brush it over the cut sides of the chicory. Place cut-sides down in a hot frying pan and cook for 2-3 minutes, turning regularly. Dress the salad and serve together.

Day 5

2 x sirtfood green juices   2 x sirtfood meals

Strawberry tabbouleh

Ingredients:

- 50g buckwheat
- 1tbsp ground turmeric
- 80g avocado
- 65g tomato
- 20g red onion
- 25g Medjool dates, pitted
- 1tbsp capers
- 30g parsley
- 100g strawberries, hulled
- 1tbsp extra virgin olive oil
- Juice 1/2 lemon
- 30g rocket

Directions:

1. Cook the buckwheat with the turmeric according to pack instructions. Drain and cool.
2. Finely chop the avocado, tomato, red onion, dates, capers and parsley and mix with the cooled buckwheat.
3. Slice the strawberries and gently mix into the salad with the oil and lemon juice. Serve on the rocket.

Miso-marinated baked cod

Ingredients:

- 20g miso
- 1tbsp mirin
- 1tbsp extra virgin olive oil
- 200g skinless cod fillet
- 20g red onion, sliced

- 40g celery, sliced
- 1 clove garlic, finely chopped
- 1 bird's eye chilli, finely chopped
- 1tsp fresh ginger, finely chopped
- 60g green beans
- 50g kale, roughly chopped
- 30g buckwheat
- 1tsp ground turmeric
- 1tsp sesame seeds
- 5g parsley, roughly chopped
- 1tbsp tamari or soy sauce

Directions:

1. Heat the oven to 220ºC/200ºC fan/gas mark 7.
2. Mix the miso, mirin and 1tsp oil, rub into the cod and marinate for 30 minutes. Transfer on to a baking tray and cook for 10 minutes.
3. Meanwhile, heat a large frying pan with the remaining oil. Add the onion and stir-fry for a few minutes, then add the celery, garlic, chilli, ginger, green beans and kale. Fry until the kale is tender and cooked through, adding a little water to soften the kale if needed.
4. Cook the buckwheat according to pack instructions with the turmeric. Add the sesame seeds, parsley and tamari or soy sauce to the stir-fry and serve with the greens and fish.

Here's how to stay motivated

Follow these top tricks and watch the pounds fall off!

A WEIGH A DAY

People who do record their weight every day are more successful losers. Download the Happy Scale app (free, iTunes) to create a chart of your progress and forecast future weight loss.

BUDDY UP

Support from others can keep you on track, and those who get diet counselling over the phone lose just as much as those who get it face-to-face.*** So if you're feeling tempted to jack it all in, have a mood-boosting mate on speed dial who can pick you back up again.

BOOST YOUR BRAIN

Tapping the chin, the inner-most point of the eyebrow and the collarbone can stop cravings, according to the Emotional Freedom Technique. Before you eat, tap each point at least seven times to curb activity in the amygdala, the part of the brain that controls the stress hormone cortisol, which is linked to increased appetite and sugar cravings.

Day 6

2 x sirtfood green juices   2 x sirtfood meals

Sirt super salad

Ingredients:

- 50g rocket
- 50g chicory leaves
- 100g smoked salmon slices
- 80g avocado, peeled, stoned and sliced
- 40g celery, sliced
- 20g red onion, sliced
- 15g walnuts, chopped
- 1tbsp capers
- 1 large Medjool date, pitted and chopped
- 1tbsp extra virgin olive oil
- Juice 1/2 lemon
- 10g parsley, chopped
- 10g lovage or celery leaves, chopped

Directions:

1. Mix all the ingredients together and serve.

Chargrilled beef

Ingredients:

- 100g potatoes, peeled and diced into 2cm cubes
- 1tbsp extra virgin olive oil
- 5g parsley, finely chopped
- 50g red onion, sliced into rings
- 50g kale, chopped
- 1 clove garlic, finely chopped
- 120-150g 3.5cm-thick beef fillet
- steak or 2cm-thick sirloin steak

- 40ml red wine
- 150ml beef stock
- 1tsp tomato purée
- 1tsp cornflour, dissolved in 1tbsp water

Directions:

1. Heat the oven to 220ºC/200ºC fan/gas mark 7.
2. Place the potatoes in a saucepan of boiling water, bring to the boil and cook for 4-5 minutes, then drain. Place in a roasting tin with 1tsp oil and cook for 35-45 minutes, turning every 10 minutes. Remove from the oven, sprinkle with the chopped parsley and mix well.
3. Fry the onion in 1tsp oil over a medium heat until soft and caramelised. Keep warm.
4. Steam the kale for 2-3 minutes, then drain. Fry the garlic gently in 1/2tsp oil for 1 minute until soft. Add the kale and fry for a further 1-2 minutes, until tender. Keep warm.
5. Heat an ovenproof frying pan until smoking. Coat the meat in 1/2tsp oil and fry according to how you like your meat done. Remove from the pan and set aside to rest. Add the wine to the hot pan to bring up any meat residue. Bubble to reduce the wine by half until it's syrupy with a concentrated flavour.
6. Add the stock and tomato purée to the steak pan and bring to the boil, then add the cornflour paste to thicken the sauce a little at a time until you have the desired consistency. Stir in any juice from the rested steak and serve with the potatoes, kale, onion rings and red wine sauce.

Day 7

2 x sirtfood green juices   2 x sirtfood meals

Sirtfood omelette

Ingredients:

- 50g streaky bacon
- 3 medium eggs
- 35g red chicory, thinly sliced
- 5g parsley, finely chopped
- 1tsp extra virgin olive oil

Directions:

1. Heat a non-stick frying pan. Cut the bacon into thin strips and cook over a high heat until crispy. You don't need to add any oil – there should be enough fat in the bacon to cook it. Remove from the pan and place on kitchen paper to drain any excess fat. Wipe the pan clean.
2. Whisk the eggs and mix with the chicory and parsley. Stir the cooked bacon through the eggs.
3. Heat the oil in a non-stick frying pan before adding the egg mixture. Cook until the omelette firms up. Ease the spatula around the edges and fold the omelette in half or roll up and serve.

Baked chicken breast

Ingredients:

For the pesto

- 15g parsley
- 15g walnuts
- 15g Parmesan
- 1tbsp extra virgin olive oil
- Juice 1/2 lemon

For the chicken

- 150g skinless chicken breast

- 20g red onions, finely sliced
- 1tsp red wine vinegar
- 35g rocket
- 100g cherry tomatoes, halved
- 1tsp balsamic vinegar

Directions:

1. Heat the oven to 220ºC/200ºC fan/gas mark 7.
2. To make the pesto, blend the parsley, walnuts, Parmesan, olive oil, half the lemon juice and 1tbsp water in a food processor until you have a smooth paste. Gradually add more water until you have your preferred consistency.
3. Marinate the chicken breast in 1tbsp of the pesto and the remaining lemon juice in the fridge for 30 minutes, or longer if possible.
4. In an ovenproof frying pan over a medium-high heat, fry the chicken in its marinade for 1 minute on either side, then transfer the pan to the oven and cook for 8 minutes, or until cooked through.
5. Marinate the onions in the red wine vinegar for 5-10 minutes, then drain off the liquid.
6. When the chicken is cooked, remove it from the oven, spoon over 1tbsp pesto and let the heat from the chicken melt the pesto. Cover with foil and leave to rest for 5 minutes before serving.
7. Combine the rocket, tomatoes and onion and drizzle over the balsamic. Serve with the chicken, spooning over the last of the pesto.

Here are nine easy Sirtfood snacks you can reach for when you need a SIRT top-up.

1 Green tea

1 cup (200ml) • 1 of your SIRT 5 a day • 0 calories

Never, ever, underestimate the healthy SIRT boost that a cup of green tea can give you. Have as many cups as you can per day – we recommend at least two cups. Not only that, the SIRTs in green tea are cumulative so you can get up to four portions of SIRTs daily if you have four cups of green tea or more.

2 Red grapes

10 grapes • 1 of your SIRT 5 a day • 30 calories

Another of the very easy Sirtfood snacks and a low-calorie way to get one of your SIRT portions. Keep a punnet or two in the fridge and have a handful at breakfast or lunch or even both!

3 Apples

1 apple • 1 of your SIRT 5 a day • 47 calories

An apple a day really does keep the doctor away. Reach for an apple as one of your after-lunch easy Sirtfood snacks. It will help keep sugar cravings at bay too.

4 Cocoa

2 tsp/10g cocoa • 1 of your SIRT 5 a day • 33 calories

Try making a chocolate shot with 2 tsp cocoa. 1 tsp sugar and 30ml milk. Mix the cocoa and sugar together with a little boiling water from the kettle to make a smooth paste. Stir in the milk. An (almost) instant chocolate hit with only 68 calories.

5 Olives

6 large black or green olives • 1 of your SIRT 5 a day • 75 calories

A versatile and easy Sirtfood snack in the afternoon or a pre-dinner treat. Serve at room temperature to get a fuller flavor.

6 Blackberries

15 blackberries • 1 of your SIRT 5 a day • 32 calories

Another of the easy Sirtfood snacks to keep in your fridge. Also great as a frozen treat.

7 Dark chocolate 85%

6 squares/20g chocolate • 1 of your SIRT 5 a day • 125 calories

Get your chocolate hit here! If you prefer 70% dark chocolate, you'll need 9 squares/30g. which will be 180 calories.

8 Pomegranate seeds

50g/half a small pack • 1 of your SIRT 5 a day • 50 calories

Easy to obtain while on the go, pomegranate seeds pack a large SIRT punch and you only need half a 100g pack to get one of your SIRT portions.

9 Blueberries

25 blueberries (80g) • 1 of your sirt 5 a day • 36 cals

One large handful of blueberries can also be one of your easy Sirtfood snacks.

10.Honey Chilli Nuts

150g (5oz) walnuts , 150g (5oz) pecan nuts , 50g (2oz) softened butter , 1 tablespoon honey

½ bird's-eye chilli, very finely chopped and de-seeded

Preheat the oven to 180C/360F. Combine the butter, honey and chilli in a bowl then add the nuts and stir them well. Spread the nuts onto a lined baking sheet and roast them in the oven for 10 minutes, stirring once halfway through. Remove from the oven and allow them to cool before eating.

Sirtfoods With Other Foods

We know that Sirtfoods and some other foods are good for us, whether its veggies like broccoli or tomatoes, spices like turmeric, or beverages like green tea. The reason these – and many other plant foods – are good for us, is primarily down to the bio-active plant compounds they contain. For the nutritionally savvy, we might be thinking of sulforaphane from broccoli, lycopene from tomatoes, curcumin from turmeric, and catechins from green tea. All the subject of extensive scientific research that goes a long way to explaining just why these foods are so good for our health.

But rather than just eating those individual foods, as good as they are, what if mixing certain foods – and therefore their nutrients – together at meals delivered an even bigger health boost? What if we could create synergies between nutrients in different foods that amplify their health benefits? It's a new idea, and here are a top-five of examples of how foods can add up for maximum effect.

1. Green tea + lemon: Green tea drinkers can expect numerous health benefits given that consuming this prized beverage is linked with less cancer, heart disease, diabetes and osteoporosis. These health benefits can be explained by its exceptional content of plant compounds called catechins, and especially a type called epigallocatechin gallate (EGCG). Adding a squeeze of lemon juice to your green tea, which is rich in vitamin C, helps to significantly increase the amount of catechins that get absorbed into the body.

2. Tomato sauce + extra virgin olive oil: Lycopene is the carotenoid responsible for the deep red color of tomatoes, and its consumption is linked with a reduced risk of certain cancers (most notably cancer of the prostate), cardiovascular disease, osteoporosis, and even protecting the skin from the damaging effects of the sun. The first thing to know about lycopene is that cooking and processing tomatoes dramatically increases the amount of lycopene that the body can absorb. The second is that the presence of fat further increases lycopene absorption. So teaming up your tomato-based dishes with a generous drizzle of extra virgin olive oil makes perfect sense.

3. Turmeric + black pepper: Turmeric, the bright yellow spice ever-present in traditional Indian cooking, is the subject of intense scientific study for its anti-cancer properties, it's potential to reduce inflammation in the body, and even for staving off dementia. This is believed to be primarily due to its active constituent curcumin. But the problem with curcumin is that it is very poorly absorbed by the body. However, adding black pepper increases its absorption, making them the perfect spice double-act. Cooking turmeric in liquid, and adding fat, further helps with curcumin absorption.

4. Broccoli + mustard: It's no secret that broccoli is good for us, with benefits including reducing cancer risk. Broccoli's main cancer-preventive ingredient is sulforaphane. This is formed when we eat broccoli by the action of an enzyme found in broccoli called myrosinase. However, cooking broccoli – especially over-cooking it – begins to destroy the myrosinase enzyme, reducing the amount of sulforaphane that can be made. In fact, if we're not careful, we can cook the benefits right out of broccoli. However, for those who like their broccoli well-cooked (rather than lightly steamed for 2 to 4 minutes), adding in other natural sources of myrosinase, such as from mustard or horseradish, means that sulforaphane can still be made.

5. Salad + avocado: Green leafy vegetables such as kale, spinach and watercress, are packed full of health-promoting carotenoids such as immune-strengthening beta-carotene and eye-friendly lutein. However, when eaten raw, in the form of salads, these carotenoids are more difficult to absorb. But the addition of some fat can really help with that and adding avocado, rich in monounsaturated fat, to a salad, has been shown to dramatically increase the number of carotenoids that can be absorbed.

Enjoy the Sirtfoods with additions and reap the added health benefits.

TURMERIC CHICKEN & KALE SALAD WITH HONEY LIME DRESSING-SIRTFOOD RECIPES

Prep time 20 mins   Cook time10 mins   Serves: 2

Ingredients

For the chicken

- 1 teaspoon ghee or 1 tbsp coconut oil
- ½ medium brown onion, diced
- 250-300 g / 9 oz. chicken mince or diced up chicken thighs
- 1 large garlic clove, finely diced
- 1 teaspoon turmeric powder
- 1teaspoon lime zest
- juice of ½ lime
- ½ teaspoon salt + pepper

For the salad

- 6 broccolini stalks or 2 cups of broccoli florets
- 2 tablespoons pumpkin seeds (pepitas)
- 3 large kale leaves, stems removed and chopped
- ½ avocado, sliced
- handful of fresh coriander leaves, chopped
- handful of fresh parsley leaves, chopped

For the dressing

- 3 tablespoons lime juice
- 1 small garlic clove, finely diced or grated
- 3 tablespoons extra-virgin olive oil (I used 1 tablespoons avocado oil and 2 tablespoons EVO)
- 1 teaspoon raw honey
- ½ teaspoon wholegrain or Dijon mustard
- ½ teaspoon sea salt and pepper

Instructions

1. Heat the ghee or coconut oil in a small frying pan over medium-high heat. Add the

onion and sauté on medium heat for 4-5 minutes, until golden. Add the chicken mince and garlic and stir for 2-3 minutes over medium-high heat, breaking it apart.

2. Add the turmeric, lime zest, lime juice, salt and pepper and cook, stirring frequently, for a further 3-4 minutes. Set the cooked mince aside.

3. While the chicken is cooking, bring a small saucepan of water to boil. Add the broccolini and cook for 2 minutes. Rinse under cold water and cut into 3-4 pieces each.

4. Add the pumpkin seeds to the frying pan from the chicken and toast over medium heat for 2 minutes, stirring frequently to prevent burning. Season with a little salt. Set aside. Raw pumpkin seeds are also fine to use.

5. Place chopped kale in a salad bowl and pour over the dressing. Using your hands, toss and massage the kale with the dressing. This will soften the kale, kind of like what citrus juice does to fish or beef carpaccio – it 'cooks' it slightly.

6. Finally toss through the cooked chicken, broccolini, fresh herbs, pumpkin seeds and avocado slices.

BUCKWHEAT NOODLES WITH CHICKEN KALE & MISO DRESSING-SIRTFOOD RECIPES

Prep time: 15 mins   Cook time: 15 mins   Serves: 2

Ingredients

For the noodles

- 2-3 handfuls of kale leaves (removed from the stem and roughly cut)
- 150 g / 5 oz buckwheat noodles (100% buckwheat, no wheat)
- 3-4 shiitake mushrooms, sliced
- 1 teaspoon coconut oil or ghee
- 1 brown onion, finely diced
- 1 medium free-range chicken breast, sliced or diced
- 1 long red chilli, thinly sliced (seeds in or out depending on how hot you like it)
- 2 large garlic cloves, finely diced
- 2-3 tablespoons Tamari sauce (gluten-free soy sauce)

For the miso dressing

- 1½ tablespoon fresh organic miso
- 1 tablespoon Tamari sauce
- 1 tablespoon extra-virgin olive oil
- 1 tablespoon lemon or lime juice
- 1 teaspoon sesame oil (optional)

Instructions

1. Bring a medium saucepan of water to boil. Add the kale and cook for 1 minute, until slightly wilted. Remove and set aside but reserve the water and bring it back to the boil. Add the soba noodles and cook according to the package instructions (usually about 5 minutes). Rinse under cold water and set aside.

2. In the meantime, pan fry the shiitake mushrooms in a little ghee or coconut oil (about a teaspoon) for 2-3 minutes, until lightly browned on each side. Sprinkle with sea salt and set aside.

3. In the same frying pan, heat more coconut oil or ghee over medium-high heat. Sauté onion and chilli for 2-3 minutes and then add the chicken pieces. Cook 5 minutes over medium heat, stirring a couple of times, then add the garlic, tamari sauce and a little

splash of water. Cook for a further 2-3 minutes, stirring frequently until chicken is cooked through.

4. Finally, add the kale and soba noodles and toss through the chicken to warm up.

5.Mix the miso dressing and drizzle over the noodles right at the end of cooking, this way you will keep all those beneficial probiotics in the miso alive and active.

ASIAN KING PRAWN STIR-FRY WITH BUCKWHEAT NOODLES –SIRTFOOD RECIPES

Serves 1

Ingredients:

- 150g shelled raw king prawns, deveined
- 2 tsp tamari (you can use soy sauce if you are not avoiding gluten)
- 2 tsp extra virgin olive oil
- 75g soba (buckwheat noodles)
- 1 garlic clove, finely chopped
- 1 bird's eye chilli, finely chopped
- 1 tsp finely chopped fresh ginger
- 20g red onions, sliced
- 40g celery, trimmed and sliced
- 75g green beans, chopped
- 50g kale, roughly chopped
- 100ml chicken stock
- 5g lovage or celery leaves

Instructions:

Heat a frying pan over a high heat, then cook the prawns in 1 teaspoon of the tamari and 1 teaspoon of the oil for 2–3 minutes. Transfer the prawns to a plate. Wipe the pan out with kitchen paper, as you're going to use it again.

Cook the noodles in boiling water for 5–8 minutes or as directed on the packet. Drain and set aside.

Meanwhile, fry the garlic, chilli and ginger, red onion, celery, beans and kale in the remaining oil over a medium–high heat for 2–3 minutes. Add the stock and bring to the boil, then simmer for a minute or two, until the vegetables are cooked but still crunchy.

Add the prawns, noodles and lovage/celery leaves to the pan, bring back to the boil then remove from the heat and serve.

BAKED SALMON SALAD WITH CREAMY MINT DRESSING-SIRTFOOD RECIPES

Serves 1   Ready in 20 minutes

Ingredients:

- 1 salmon fillet (130g)
- 40g mixed salad leaves
- 40g young spinach leaves
- 2 radishes, trimmed and thinly sliced
- 5cm piece (50g) cucumber, cut into chunks
- 2 spring onions, trimmed and sliced
- 1 small handful (10g) parsley, roughly chopped

For the dressing:

- 1 tsp low-fat mayonnaise
- 1 tbsp natural yogurt
- 1 tbsp rice vinegar
- 2 leaves mint, finely chopped
- Salt and freshly ground black pepper

Instructions:

1 Preheat the oven to 200°C (180°C fan/Gas 6).

2 Place the salmon fillet on a baking tray and bake for 16–18 minutes until just cooked through. Remove from the oven and set aside. The salmon is equally nice hot or cold in the salad. If your salmon has skin, simply cook skin side down and remove the salmon from the skin using a fish slice after cooking. It should slide off easily when cooked.

3 In a small bowl, mix together the mayonnaise, yogurt, rice wine vinegar, mint leaves

and salt and pepper together and leave to stand for at least 5 minutes to allow the flavors to develop.

4 Arrange the salad leaves and spinach on a serving plate and top with the radishes, cucumber, spring onions and parsley. Flake the cooked salmon onto the salad and drizzle the dressing over.

CHOC CHIP GRANOLA-SIRTFOOD RECIPES

244 calories   Serves 8   Ready in 30 minutes

Ingredients:

- 200g jumbo oats
- 50g pecans, roughly
- chopped
- 3 tbsp light olive oil
- 20g butter
- 1 tbsp dark brown sugar
- 2 tbsp rice malt syrup
- 60g good-quality (70%)
- dark chocolate chips

Instructions:

1 Preheat the oven to 160°C (140°C fan/Gas 3). Line a large baking tray with a silicone sheet or baking parchment.

2 Mix the oats and pecans together in a large bowl. In a small non-stick pan, gently heat the olive oil, butter, brown sugar and rice malt syrup until the butter has melted and the sugar and syrup have dissolved. Do not allow to boil. Pour the syrup over the oats and stir thoroughly until the oats are fully covered.

3 Distribute the granola over the baking tray, spreading right into the corners. Leave clumps of mixture with spacing rather than an even spread. Bake in the oven for 20 minutes until just tinged golden brown at the edges. Remove from the oven and leave to cool on the tray completely.

4 When cool, break up any bigger lumps on the tray with your fingers and then mix in the chocolate chips. Scoop or pour the granola into an airtight tub or jar. The granola will keep for at least 2 weeks.

FRAGRANT ASIAN HOTPOT-SIRTFOOD RECIPES

185 calories   Serves 2   Ready in 15 minutes

Ingredients:

- 1 tsp tomato purée
- 1 star anise, crushed (or 1/4 tsp ground anise)
- Small handful (10g) parsley, stalks finely chopped
- Small handful (10g) coriander, stalks finely chopped
- Juice of 1/2 lime
- 500ml chicken stock, fresh or made with 1 cube
- 1/2 carrot, peeled and cut into matchsticks
- 50g broccoli, cut into small florets
- 50g beansprouts
- 100g raw tiger prawns
- 100g firm tofu, chopped
- 50g rice noodles, cooked according to packet instructions
- 50g cooked water chestnuts, drained
- 20g sushi ginger, chopped
- 1 tbsp good-quality miso paste

Instructions:

Place the tomato purée, star anise, parsley stalks, coriander stalks, lime juice and chicken stock in a large pan and bring to a simmer for 10 minutes.

Add the carrot, broccoli, prawns, tofu, noodles and water chestnuts and simmer gently until the prawns are cooked through. Remove from the heat and stir in the sushi ginger and miso paste.

Serve sprinkled with the parsley and coriander leaves.

LAMB,BUTTERNUT SQUASH AND DATE TAGINE-SIRTFOOD RECIPES

Prep time15 mins   Cook time1 hour 15 mins   Serves: 4

Ingredients

- 2 tablespoons olive oil
- 1 red onion, sliced
- 2cm ginger, grated
- 3 garlic cloves, grated or crushed
- 1 teaspoon chilli flakes (or to taste)
- 2 teaspoons cumin seeds
- 1 cinnamon stick
- 2 teaspoons ground turmeric
- 800g lamb neck fillet, cut into 2cm chunks
- ½ teaspoon salt
- 100g medjool dates, pitted and chopped
- 400g tin chopped tomatoes, plus half a can of water
- 500g butternut squash, chopped into 1cm cubes
- 400g tin chickpeas, drained
- 2 tablespoons fresh coriander (plus extra for garnish)
- Buckwheat, couscous, flatbreads or rice to serve

INSTRUCTIONS:

1.Preheat your oven to 140C.

2.Drizzle about 2 tablespoons of olive oil into a large ovenproof saucepan or cast iron casserole dish. Add the sliced onion and cook on a gentle heat, with the lid on, for about 5 minutes, until the onions are softened but not brown.

3.Add the grated garlic and ginger, chilli, cumin, cinnamon and turmeric. Stir well and cook for 1 more minute with the lid off. Add a splash of water if it gets too dry.

4.Next add in the lamb chunks. Stir well to coat the meat in the onions and spices and then add the salt, chopped dates and tomatoes, plus about half a can of water (100-200ml).

5.Bring the tagine to the boil and then put the lid on and put in your preheated oven for 1 hour and 15 minutes.

6.Thirty minutes before the end of the cooking time, add in the chopped butternut squash and drained chickpeas. Stir everything together, put the lid back on and return to the oven for the final 30 minutes of cooking.

7.When the tagine is ready, remove from the oven and stir through the chopped coriander. Serve with buckwheat, couscous, flatbreads or basmati rice.

Notes

If you don't own an ovenproof saucepan or cast iron casserole dish, simply cook the tagine in a regular saucepan up until it has to go in the oven and then transfer the tagine into a regular lidded casserole dish before placing in the oven. Add on an extra 5 minutes cooking time to allow for the fact that the casserole dish will need extra time to heat up.

TURMERIC BAKED SALMON-SIRTFOOD RECIPES

Serves: 1   Preparation time:10 – 15 minutes   Cooking time:10 minutes

Ingredients

- 125-150 g Skinned Salmon
- 1 tsp Extra virgin olive oil
- 1 tsp Ground turmeric
- 1/4 Juice of a lemon
- For the spicy celery
- 1 tsp Extra virgin olive oil
- 40 g Red onion, finely chopped
- 60 g Tinned green lentils
- 1 Garlic clove, finely chopped
- 1 cm Fresh ginger, finely chopped
- 1 Bire's eye chilli, finely chopped
- 150 g Celery, cut into 2cm lengths
- 1 tsp Mild curry powder
- 130 g Tomato, cut into 8 wedges
- 100 ml Chicken or vegetable stock
- 1 tbsp Chopped parsley

INSTRUCTIONS:

1.Heat the oven to 200C / gas mark 6.

Start with the spicy celery. Heat a frying pan over a medium–low heat, add the olive oil, then the onion, garlic, ginger, chilli and celery. Fry gently for 2–3 minutes or until softened but not coloured, then add the curry powder and cook for a further minute.

2.Add the tomatoes then the stock and lentils and simmer gently for 10 minutes. You may want to increase or decrease the cooking time depending on how crunchy you like your celery.

3.Meanwhile, mix the turmeric, oil and lemon juice and rub over the salmon. # Place on a baking tray and cook for 8–10 minutes.

4.To finish, stir the parsley through the celery and serve with the salmon.

CORONATION CHICKEN SALAD-SIRTFOOD RECIPES

Serves 1   Preparation time: 5 minutes

Ingredients

- 75 g Natural yoghurt
- Juice of 1/4 of a lemon
- 1 tsp Coriander, chopped
- 1 tsp Ground turmeric
- 1/2 tsp Mild curry powder
- 100 g Cooked chicken breast, cut into bite-sized pieces
- 6 Walnut halves, finely chopped
- 1 Medjool date, finely chopped
- 20 g Red onion, diced
- 1 Bird's eye chilli
- 40 g Rocket, to serve

INSTRUCTIONS:

Mix the yoghurt, lemon juice, coriander and spices together in a bowl. Add all the remaining ingredients and serve on a bed of the rocket.

BAKED POTATOES WITH SPICY CHICKPEA STEW-SIRTFOOD RECIPES

Prep time10 mins   Cook time1 hour   Serves 4-6

Ingredients

- 4-6 baking potatoes, pricked all over
- 2 tablespoons olive oil
- 2 red onions, finely chopped
- 4 cloves garlic, grated or crushed
- 2cm ginger, grated
- ½ -2 teaspoons chilli flakes (depending on how hot you like things)
- 2 tablespoons cumin seeds
- 2 tablespoons turmeric
- Splash of water
- 2 x 400g tins chopped tomatoes
- 2 tablespoons unsweetened cocoa powder (or cacao)
- 2 x 400g tins chickpeas (or kidney beans if you prefer) including the chickpea water DON'T DRAIN!!
- 2 yellow peppers (or whatever colour you prefer!), chopped into bitesize pieces
- 2 tablespoons parsley plus extra for garnish
- Salt and pepper to taste (optional)
- Side salad (optional)

INSTRUCTIONS:

1.Preheat the oven to 200C, meanwhile you can prepare all your ingredients.

2.When the oven is hot enough put your baking potatoes in the oven and cook for 1 hour or until they are done how you like them.

3.Once the potatoes are in the oven, place the olive oil and chopped red onion in a large wide saucepan and cook gently, with the lid on for 5 minutes, until the onions are soft but not brown.

4.Remove the lid and add the garlic, ginger, cumin and chilli. Cook for a further minute on a low heat, then add the turmeric and a very small splash of water and cook for another minute, taking care not to let the pan get too dry.

5.Next, add in the tomatoes, cocoa powder (or cacao), chickpeas (including the chickpea water) and yellow pepper. Bring to the boil, then simmer on a low heat for 45 minutes until the sauce is thick and unctuous (but don't let it burn!). The stew should be done at roughly the same time as the potatoes.

6.Finally stir in the 2 tablespoons of parsley, and some salt and pepper if you wish, and serve the stew on top of the baked potatoes, perhaps with a simple side salad.

KALE AND RED ONION DHAL WITH BUCKWHEAT-SIRTFOOD RECIPES

Prep time5 mins   Cook time25 mins   Serves:4

INGREDIENTS

- 1 tablespoon olive oil
- 1 small red onion, sliced
- 3 garlic cloves, grated or crushed
- 2 cm ginger, grated
- 1 birds eye chilli, deseeded and finely chopped (more if you like things hot!)
- 2 teaspoons turmeric
- 2 teaspoons garam masala
- 160g red lentils
- 400ml coconut milk
- 200ml water
- 100g kale (or spinach would be a great alternative)
- 160g buckwheat (or brown rice)

INSTRUCTIONS:

1.Put the olive oil in a large, deep saucepan and add the sliced onion. Cook on a low heat, with the lid on for 5 minutes until softened.

2.Add the garlic, ginger and chilli and cook for 1 more minute.

3.Add the turmeric, garam masala and a splash of water and cook for 1 more minute.

4.Add the red lentils, coconut milk, and 200ml water (do this simply by half filling the coconut milk can with water and tipping it into the saucepan).

5.Mix everything together thoroughly and cook for 20 minutes over a gently heat with the lid on. Stir occasionally and add a little more water if the dhal starts to stick.

6.After 20 minutes add the kale, stir thoroughly and replace the lid, cook for a further 5 minutes (1-2 minutes if you use spinach instead!)

7.About 15 minutes before the curry is ready, place the buckwheat in a medium saucepan and add plenty of boiling water. Bring the water back to the boil and cook for 10 minutes (or a little longer if you prefer your buckwheat softer. Drain the buckwheat in a sieve and serve with the dhal.

CHARGRILLED BEEF WITH A RED WINE JUS, ONION RINGS, GARLIC KALE AND HERB ROASTED POTATOES-SIRTFOOD RECIPES

INGREDIENTS:

- 100g potatoes, peeled and cut into 2cm dice
- 1 tbsp extra virgin olive oil
- 5g parsley, finely chopped
- 50g red onion, sliced into rings
- 50g kale, sliced
- 1 garlic clove, finely chopped
- 120–150g x 3.5cm-thick beef fillet steak or 2cm-thick sirloin steak
- 40ml red wine
- 150ml beef stock
- 1 tsp tomato purée
- 1 tsp cornflour, dissolved in 1 tbsp water

INSTRUCTIONS:

Heat the oven to 220ºC/gas 7.

Place the potatoes in a saucepan of boiling water, bring back to the boil and cook for 4–5 minutes, then drain. Place in a roasting tin with 1 teaspoon of the oil and roast in the hot oven for 35–45 minutes. Turn the potatoes every 10 minutes to ensure even cooking. When cooked, remove from the oven, sprinkle with the chopped parsley and mix well.

Fry the onion in 1 teaspoon of the oil over a medium heat for 5–7 minutes, until soft and nicely caramelised. Keep warm. Steam the kale for 2–3 minutes then drain. Fry the garlic gently in ½ teaspoon of oil for 1 minute, until soft but not coloured. Add the kale and fry for a further 1–2 minutes, until tender. Keep warm.

Heat an ovenproof frying pan over a high heat until smoking. Coat the meat in ½ a teaspoon of the oil and fry in the hot pan over a medium–high heat according to how you like your meat done.If you like your meat medium it would be better to sear the meat and then transfer the pan to an oven set at 220ºC/gas 7 and finish the cooking that way for the prescribed times.

Remove the meat from the pan and set aside to rest. Add the wine to the hot pan to bring up any meat residue. Bubble to reduce the wine by half, until syrupy and with a concentrated flavor.

Add the stock and tomato purée to the steak pan and bring to the boil, then add the cornflour paste to thicken your sauce, adding it a little at a time until you have your desired consistency. Stir in any of the juices from the rested steak and serve with the roasted potatoes, kale, onion rings and red wine sauce.

KALE AND BLACKCURRANT SMOOTHIE-SIRTFOOD RECIPES

86 calories   Serves 2   Ready in 3 minutes

INGREDIENTS:

- 2 tsp honey
- 1 cup freshly made green tea
- 10 baby kale leaves, stalks removed
- 1 ripe banana
- 40 g blackcurrants, washed and stalks removed
- 6 ice cubes

INSTRUCTIONS:

Stir the honey into the warm green tea until dissolved. Whiz all the ingredients together in a blender until smooth. Serve immediately.

BUCKWHEAT PASTA SALAD-SIRTFOOD RECIPES

Serves 1

INGREDIENTS:

- 50g buckwheat pasta(cooked according to the packet instructions)
- large handful of rocket
- small handful of basil leaves
- 8 cherry tomatoes,halved
- 1/2 avocado,diced
- 10 olives
- 1 tbsp extra virgin olive oil
- 20g pine nuts

Directions:

Gently combine all the ingredients except the pine nuts and arrange on a plate or in a bowl,then scatter the pine nuts over the top.

GREEK SALAD SKEWERS-SIRTFOOD RECIPES

306 calories   Serves 2   Ready in 10 minutes

INGREDIENTS:

- 2 wooden skewers, soaked in water for 30 minutes before use
- 8 large black olives
- 8 cherry tomatoes
- 1 yellow pepper, cut into 8 squares
- ½ red onion, cut in half and separated into 8 pieces
- 100g (about 10cm) cucumber, cut into 4 slices and halved
- 100g feta, cut into 8 cubes

For the dressing:

- 1 tbsp extra virgin olive oil
- Juice of ½ lemon
- 1 tsp balsamic vinegar

- ½ clove garlic, peeled and crushed
- Few leaves basil, finely chopped (or ½ tsp dried mixed herbs to replace basil and oregano)
- Few leaves oregano, finely chopped
- Generous seasoning of salt and freshly ground black pepper

INSTRUCTIONS:

1 Thread each skewer with the salad ingredients in the order: olive, tomato, yellow pepper, red onion, cucumber, feta, tomato, olive, yellow pepper, red onion, cucumber, feta.

2 Place all the dressing ingredients in a small bowl and mix together thoroughly. Pour over the skewers.

KALE, EDAMAME AND TOFU CURRY-SIRTFOOD RECIPES

342 calories   Serves 4   Ready in 45 minutes

INGREDIENTS:

- 1 tbsp rapeseed oil
- 1 large onion, chopped
- 4 cloves garlic, peeled and grated
- 1 large thumb (7cm) fresh ginger, peeled and grated
- 1 red chilli, deseeded and thinly sliced
- 1/2 tsp ground turmeric
- 1/4 tsp cayenne pepper
- 1 tsp paprika
- 1/2 tsp ground cumin
- 1 tsp salt
- 250g dried red lentils
- 1 litre boiling water
- 50g frozen soyaedamame beans
- 200g firm tofu, chopped into cubes
- 2 tomatoes, roughly chopped
- Juice of 1 lime

- 200g kale leaves, stalks removed and torn

INSTRUCTIONS:

1 Put the oil in a heavy-bottomed pan over a low-medium heat. Add the onion and cook for 5 minutes before adding the garlic, ginger and chilli and cooking for a further 2 minutes. Add the turmeric, cayenne, paprika, cumin and salt. Stir through before adding the red lentils and stirring again.

2 Pour in the boiling water and bring to a hearty simmer for 10 minutes, then reduce the heat and cook for a further 20-30 minutes until the curry has a thick '•porridge' consistency.

3 Add the soya beans, tofu and tomatoes and cook for a further 5 minutes. Add the lime juice and kale leaves and cook until the kale is just tender.

CHOCOLATE CUPCAKES WITH MATCHA ICING-SIRTFOOD RECIPES

234 calories   MAKES 12   READY IN 35 MINUTES

INGREDIENTS:

- 150g self-raising flour
- 200g caster sugar
- 60g cocoa
- ½ tsp salt
- ½ tsp fine espresso coffee, decaf if preferred
- 120ml milk
- ½ tsp vanilla extract
- 50ml vegetable oil
- 1 egg
- 120ml boiling water

For the icing:

- 50g butter, at room temperature
- 50g icing sugar
- 1 tbsp matcha green tea powder
- ½ tsp vanilla bean paste

- 50g soft cream cheese

INSTRUCTIONS:

Preheat the oven to 180C/160C fan. Line a cupcake tin with paper or silicone cake cases.

Place the flour, sugar, cocoa, salt and espresso powder in a large bowl and mix thoroughly.

Add the milk, vanilla extract, vegetable oil and egg to the dry ingredients and use an electric mixer to beat until well combined. Carefully pour in the boiling water slowly and beat on a low speed until fully combined. Use a high speed to beat for a further minute to add air to the batter. The batter is much more liquid than a normal cake mix. Have faith, it will taste amazing!

Spoon the batter evenly between the cake cases. Each cake case should be no more than ¾ full. Bake in the oven for 15-18 minutes, until the mixture bounces back when tapped. Remove from the oven and allow to cool completely before icing.

To make the icing, cream the butter and icing sugar together until it's pale and smooth. Add the matcha powder and vanilla and stir again. Finally add the cream cheese and beat until smooth. Pipe or spread over the cakes.

SESAME CHICKEN SALAD-Sirtfood Recipes

304 cals   Serves 2   Ready in 12 minutes

INGREDIENTS:

- 1 tbsp sesame seeds
- 1 cucumber, peeled, halved lengthways, deseeded with a teaspoon and sliced
- 100g baby kale, roughly chopped
- 60g pak choi, very finely shredded
- ½ red onion, very finely sliced
- Large handful (20g) parsley, chopped
- 150g cooked chicken, shredded

For the dressing:

- 1 tbsp extra virgin olive oil
- 1 tsp sesame oil
- Juice of 1 lime
- 1 tsp clear honey
- 2 tsp soy sauce

INSTRUCTIONS:

1 Toast the sesame seeds in a dry frying pan for 2 minutes until lightly browned and fragrant. Transfer to a plate to cool.

2 In a small bowl, mix together the olive oil, sesame oil, lime juice, honey and soy sauce to make the dressing.

3 Place the cucumber, kale, pak choi, red onion and parsley in a large bowl and gently mix together. Pour over the dressing and mix again.

4 Distribute the salad between two plates and top with the shredded chicken. Sprinkle over the sesame seeds just before serving.

SirtFood Mushroom Scramble Eggs-Sirtfood Recipes

Ingredients

- 2 eggs
- 1 tsp ground turmeric
- 1 tsp mild curry powder
- 20g kale, roughly chopped
- 1 tsp extra virgin olive oil
- ½ bird's eye chilli, thinly sliced
- handful of button mushrooms, thinly sliced
- 5g parsley, finely chopped
- Add a seed mixture as a topper and some Rooster Sauce for flavor *optional*

Instructions

1. Mix the turmeric and curry powder and add a little water until you have achieved a light paste.
2. Steam the kale for 2– 3 minutes.
3. Heat the oil in a frying pan over a medium heat and fry the chilli and mushrooms for 2– 3 minutes until they have started to brown and soften.

Aromatic Chicken Breast with Kale, Red Onion, and Salsa-Sirtfood Recipes

Ingredients:

- 120g skinless, boneless chicken breast
- 2 tsp ground turmeric
- juice of ¼ lemon
- 1 tbsp extra virgin olive oil
- 50g kale, chopped
- 20g red onion, sliced
- 1 tsp chopped fresh ginger
- 50g buckwheat

Instructions:

1. To make the salsa, remove the eye from the tomato and chop it very finely,

taking care to keep as much of the liquid as possible. Mix with the chilli, capers, parsley and lemon juice. You could put everything in a blender but the end result is a little different.

2. Heat the oven to 220ºC/gas 7. Marinate the chicken breast in 1 teaspoon of the turmeric, the lemon juice and a little oil. Leave for 5–10 minutes.

3. Heat an ovenproof frying pan until hot, then add the marinated chicken and cook for a minute or so on each side, until pale golden, then transfer to the oven (place on a baking tray if your pan isn't ovenproof) for 8–10 minutes or until cooked through. Remove from the oven, cover with foil and leave to rest for 5 minutes before serving.

4. Meanwhile, cook the kale in a steamer for 5 minutes. Fry the red onions and the ginger in a little oil, until soft but not coloured, then add the cooked kale and fry for another minute.

5. Cook the buckwheat according to the packet instructions with the remaining teaspoon of turmeric. Serve alongside the chicken, vegetables and salsa.

Smoked Salmon Omelette

Serves:1   Preparation time:5 – 10 minutes

Ingredients

- 2 Medium eggs
- 100 g Smoked salmon, sliced
- 1/2 tsp Capers
- 10 g Rocket, chopped
- 1 tsp Parsley, chopped
- 1 tsp Extra virgin olive oil

Instructions:

1. Crack the eggs into a bowl and whisk well. Add the salmon, capers, rocket and parsley.
2. Heat the olive oil in a non-stick frying pan until hot but not smoking. Add the egg mixture and, using a spatula or fish slice, move the mixture around the pan until it is even. Reduce the heat and let the omelette cook through. Slide the spatula around the edges and roll up or fold the omelette in half to serve.

Green Tea Smoothie-Sirtfood Recipes

Serves 2   Ready in 3 minutes

Ingredients

- 2 ripe bananas
- 250 ml milk
- 2 tsp matcha green tea powder
- 1/2 tsp vanilla bean paste (not extract) or a small scrape of the seeds from a vanilla pod
- 6 ice cubes
- 2 tsp honey

Instructions:

Simply blend all the ingredients together in a blender and serve in two glasses.

SIRT FOOD MISO MARINATED COD WITH STIR FRIED GREENS & SESAME-SIRTFOOD RECIPES

SERVES 1

INGREDIENTS

- 20g miso
- 1 tbsp mirin
- 1 tbsp extra virgin olive oil
- 200g skinless cod fillet
- 20g red onion, sliced
- 40g celery, sliced
- 1 garlic clove, finely chopped
- 1 bird's eye chilli, finely chopped
- 1 tsp finely chopped fresh ginger
- 60g green beans
- 50g kale, roughly chopped

- 1 tsp sesame seeds
- 5g parsley, roughly chopped
- 1 tbsp tamari
- 30g buckwheat
- 1 tsp ground turmeric

INSTRUCTIONS

1. Mix the miso, mirin and 1 teaspoon of the oil. Rub all over the cod and leave to marinate for 30 minutes. Heat the oven to 220ºC/gas 7.
2. Bake the cod for 10 minutes.
3. Meanwhile, heat a large frying pan or wok with the remaining oil. Add the onion and stir-fry for a few minutes, then add the celery, garlic, chilli, ginger, green beans and kale. Toss and fry until the kale is tender and cooked through. You may need to add a little water to the pan to aid the cooking process.
4. Cook the buckwheat according to the packet instructions with the turmeric for 3 minutes.
5. Add the sesame seeds, parsley and tamari to the stir-fry and serve with the greens and fish.

Raspberry and Blackcurrant Jelly-Sirtfood Recipes

Serves 2   Ready in 15 minutes + setting time

INGREDIENTS

- 100g raspberries, washed
- 2 leaves gelatine
- 100g blackcurrants, washed and stalks removed
- 2 tbsp granulated sugar
- 300ml water

INSTRUCTIONS

1 Arrange the raspberries in two serving dishes/glasses/moulds. Put the gelatine leaves in a bowl of cold water to soften.

2 Place the blackcurrants in a small pan with the sugar and 100ml water and bring to

the boil. Simmer vigorously for 5 minutes and then remove from the heat. Leave to stand for 2 minutes.

3 Squeeze out excess water from the gelatine leaves and add them to the saucepan. Stir until fully dissolved, then stir in the rest of the water. Pour the liquid into the prepared dishes and refrigerate to set. The jellies should be ready in about 3-4 hours or overnight.

Apple Pancakes with Blackcurrant Compote-Sirtfood Recipes

Serves 4   Ready in 20 minutes

INGREDIENTS

- 75g porridge oats
- 125g plain flour
- 1 tsp baking powder
- 2 tbsp caster sugar
- Pinch of salt
- 2 apples, peeled, cored and cut into small pieces
- 300ml semi-skimmed milk
- 2 egg whites
- 2 tsp light olive oil

For the compote:

- 120g blackcurrants, washed and stalks removed
- 2 tbsp caster sugar
- 3 tbsp water

Directions:

1 First make the compote. Place the blackcurrants, sugar and water in a small pan. Bring up to a simmer and cook for 10-15 minutes.

2 Place the oats, flour, baking powder, caster sugar and salt in a large bowl and mix well. Stir in the apple and then whisk in the milk a little at a time until you have a smooth mixture. Whisk the egg whites to stiff peaks and then fold into the pancake batter. Transfer the batter to a jug.

3 Heat 1/2 tsp oil in a non-stick frying pan on a medium-high heat and pour in approximately one quarter of the batter. Cook on both sides until golden brown. Remove and repeat to make four pancakes.

4 Serve the pancakes with the blackcurrant compote drizzled over.

SIRT Fruit Salad- Sirtfood Recipes

This fruit salad is packed full of the best fruit SIRTs.

Serves 1   Ready in 10 minutes

INGREDIENTS

- ½ cup freshly made green tea
- 1 tsp honey
- 1 orange, halved
- 1 apple, cored and roughly chopped
- 10 red seedless grapes
- 10 blueberries

Directions:

1 Stir the honey into half a cup of green tea. When dissolved, add the juice of half the orange. Leave to cool.

2 Chop the other half of the orange and place in a bowl together with the chopped apple, grapes and blueberries. Pour over the cooled tea and leave to steep for a few minutes before serving.

SIRTFOOD BITES-SIRTFOOD RECIPES

INGREDIENTS

- 120g walnuts
- 30g dark chocolate (85 per cent cocoa solids), broken into pieces; or cocoa nibs
- 250g Medjool dates, pitted
- 1 tbsp cocoa powder
- 1 tbsp ground turmeric
- 1 tbsp extra virgin olive oil
- the scraped seeds of one vanilla pod or 1 tsp vanilla extract
- 1–2 tbsp water

Directions:

1. Place the walnuts and chocolate in a food processor and process until you have a fine powder.
2. Add all the other ingredients except the water and blend until the mixture forms a ball. You may or may not have to add the water depending on the consistency of the mixture – you don't want it to be too sticky.
3. Using your hands, form the mixture into bite-sized balls and refrigerate in an airtight container for at least one hour before eating them.
4. You could roll some of the balls in some more cocoa or desiccated coconut to achieve a different finish if you like.
5. They will keep for up to one week in your fridge.

SIRT MUESLI-SIRTFOOD RECIPES

Ingredients:

- 20g buckwheat flakes
- 10g buckwheat puffs
- 15g coconut flakes or desiccated coconut
- 40g Medjool dates, pitted and chopped
- 15g walnuts, chopped
- 10g cocoa nibs
- 100g strawberries, hulled and chopped
- 100g plain Greek yoghurt (or vegan alternative, such as soya or coconut yoghurt)

Instructions:

Mix all of the above ingredients together, only adding the yoghurt and strawberries before serving if you are making it in bulk.

CHINESE-STYLE PORK WITH PAK CHOI-SIRTFOOD RECIPES

Ingredients

- 400g firm tofu, cut into large cubes
- 1 tbsp cornflour
- 1 tbsp water
- 125ml chicken stock
- 1 tbsp rice wine
- 1 tbsp tomato purée
- 1 tsp brown sugar
- 1 tbsp soy sauce
- 1 clove garlic, peeled and crushed
- 1 thumb (5cm) fresh ginger, peeled and grated 1 tbsp rapeseed oil
- 100g shiitake mushrooms, sliced
- 1 shallot, peeled and sliced
- 200g pak choi or choi sum, cut into thin slices 400g pork mince (10% fat)
- 100g beansprouts
- Large handful (20g) parsley, chopped

Instructions:

1. Lay out the tofu on kitchen paper, cover with more kitchen paper and set aside.
2. In a small bowl, mix together the cornflour and water, removing all lumps. Add the chicken stock, rice wine, tomato purée, brown sugar and soy sauce. Add the crushed garlic and ginger and stir together.
3. In a wok or large frying pan, heat the oil to a high temperature. Add the shiitake mushrooms and stir-fry for 2–3 minutes until cooked and glossy. Remove the mushrooms from the pan with a slotted spoon and set aside. Add the tofu to the pan and stir-fry until golden on all sides. Remove with a slotted spoon and set aside.
4. Add the shallot and pak choi to the wok, stir-fry for 2 minutes, then add the mince. Cook until the mince is cooked through, then add the sauce, reduce the heat a notch and allow the sauce to bubble round the meat for a minute or two. Add the beansprouts, shiitake mushrooms and tofu to the pan and warm through. Remove from the heat, stir through the parsley and serve immediately.

Tuscan Bean Stew-Sirtfood Recipes

Ingredients

- 1 tbsp extra virgin olive oil
- 50g red onion, finely chopped
- 30g carrot, peeled and finely chopped
- 30g celery, trimmed and finely chopped
- 1 garlic clove, finely chopped
- ½ bird's eye chilli, finely chopped (optional)
- 1 tsp herbes de Provence
- 200ml vegetable stock
- 1 x 400g tin chopped Italian tomatoes
- 1 tsp tomato purée
- 200g tinned mixed beans
- 50g kale, roughly chopped
- 1 tbsp roughly chopped parsley
- 40g buckwheat

Directions:

Place the oil in a medium saucepan over a low–medium heat and gently fry the onion, carrot, celery, garlic, chilli(if using) and herbs, until the onion is soft but not colored.

Add the stock, tomatoes and tomato purée and bring to the boil. Add the beans and simmer for 30 minutes.

Add the kale and cook for another 5–10 minutes, until tender, then add the parsley.

Meanwhile, cook the buckwheat according to the packet instructions, drain and then serve with the stew.

Salmon Sirt Super Salad-Sirtfood Recipes

Makes 1

Ingredients

- 50g rocket
- 50g chicory leaves
- 100g smoked salmon slices (you can also use lentils, cooked chicken breast or tinned tuna)
- 80g avocado, peeled, stoned and sliced
- 40g celery, sliced
- 20g red onion, sliced
- 15g walnuts, chopped
- 1 tbs capers
- 1 large Medjool date, pitted and chopped
- 1 tbs extra-virgin olive oil
- Juice ¼ lemon
- 10g parsley, chopped
- 10g lovage or celery leaves, chopped

Directions:

Arrange the salad leaves on a large plate. Mix all the remaining ingredients together and serve on top of the leaves.

CHAPTER 14: BREAKFAST RECIPES
Dark Chocolate Granola

Ingredients:

- 1 c. whole oats
- ¼ c. raw walnuts, chopped
- ¼ c. good quality dark chocolate chips (at least 70% cacao)
- 3 Tbsp. light olive oil
- 2 Tbsp. rice malt syrup
- 1 Tbsp. brown sugar
- 1 Tbsp. butter

Directions:

1. Preheat the oven to 325 degrees.

2. Line a cookie sheet with parchment paper or silicone sheet.

3. Mix the oats and walnuts in a large bowl.

4. In a small pot, combine the olive oil, malt syrup, brown sugar, and butter. Heat over medium heat until the sugar has dissolved and the butter has melted, but do not let it boil.

5. Pour the heated mixture over the oats and stir until the oats are completely coated.

6. Pour the oats onto the cookie sheet and spread them evenly. Bake them for 20 minutes, or until the oats turn golden brown around the edges.

7. Allow to cool thoroughly.

8. Use your fingers to break up the granola, then mix in the chocolate chips and transfer to an air-tight jar.

Sirtfood Fruit Salad

Ingredients:

- 1 medium green apple, cored and roughly chopped
- 1 orange, cut in half
- 10 red grapes
- 10 blueberries
- ½ c. freshly brewed green tea
- 1 tsp. raw honey

Directions:

1. Combine the apple, grapes, and blueberries in a bowl.

2. Squeeze the juice of one half of the orange into the fruit.

3. Chop the other half of the orange and add the fruit to the bowl.

4. Stir the honey into the green tea and allow it to dissolve.

5. Pour the tea over the fruit, and enjoy immediately.

Strawberry Buckwheat Pancakes

Ingredients

- 100g (3½oz) strawberries, chopped
- 100g (3½ oz) buckwheat flour
- 1 egg
- 250mls (8fl oz) milk
- 1 teaspoon olive oil
- 1 teaspoon olive oil for frying
- Freshly squeezed juice of 1 orange

Directions:

Pour the milk into a bowl and mix in the egg and a teaspoon of olive oil. Sift in the flour to the liquid mixture until smooth and creamy. Allow it to rest for 15 minutes. Heat a little oil in a pan and pour in a quarter of the mixture (or to the size you prefer.) Sprinkle in a quarter of the strawberries into the batter. Cook for around 2 minutes on each side. Serve hot with a drizzle of orange juice. You could try experimenting with other berries such as blueberries and blackberries.

Blackcurrant and Kale Breakfast Smoothie

Ingredients:

- 1 ripe banana
- ¼ c. blackcurrants
- 10 baby kale leaves, stems removed
- 1 c. freshly made green tea
- 2 tsp. honey
- 6 ice cubes

Directions:

1. Stir the honey into the warm green tea until it is completely dissolved.

2. Add all ingredients to the blender and blend until smooth.

3. This recipe is easy to double if you have more than one person in your family doing The Sirtfood Diet.

Green Sirtfood Omelet

Ingredients:

- 2 large eggs at room temperature
- 1 handful of arugula
- 2 Tbsp. chopped flat leaf parsley
- 1 Tbsp. chopped red onion
- 1 Tbsp. olive oil

Directions:

1. Put the olive oil into a large frying pan and heat it gently.

2. Add the onion and cook over low heat for approximately five minutes, or until the onion is translucent.

3. Beat the two eggs in a bowl.

4. Spread the onions out evenly over the pan before pouring the eggs into the pan.

5. Cook for one or two minutes until the eggs begin to set at the edges, then lift the edges, and let the uncooked eggs run underneath the cooked eggs.

6. Add the arugula and parsley to the top of the eggs.

7. Continue cooking until the eggs are nearly set. Fold the omelet in half and continue cooking for one more minute.

8. Transfer to a plate and enjoy.

Matcha Green Juice

Preparation time: 10 minutes   Servings: 2

Ingredients:

- 5 ounces fresh kale
- 2 ounces fresh arugula
- ¼ cup fresh parsley
- 4 celery stalks
- 1 green apple, cored and chopped
- 1 (1-inch) piece fresh ginger, peeled
- 1 lemon, peeled
- ½ teaspoon matcha green tea

Directions:

1. Add all ingredients into a juicer and extract the juice according to the manufacturer's method.
2. Pour into 2 glasses and serve immediately.

Celery Juice

Preparation time: 10 minutes   Servings: 2

Ingredients:

- 8 celery stalks with leaves
- 2 tablespoons fresh ginger, peeled
- 1 lemon, peeled
- ½ cup filtered water
- Pinch of salt

Directions:

Place all the ingredients in a blender and pulse until well combined.

Through a fine mesh strainer, strain the juice and transfer into 2 glasses.

Serve immediately.

Kale & Orange Juice

Preparation time: 10 minutes   Servings: 2

Ingredients:

- 5 large oranges, peeled and sectioned
- 2 bunches fresh kale

Directions:

1. Add all ingredients into a juicer and extract the juice according to the manufacturer's method.
2. Pour into 2 glasses and serve immediately.

Apple & Cucumber Juice

Preparation time: 10 minutes   Servings: 2

Ingredients:

- 3 large apples, cored and sliced
- 2 large cucumbers, sliced
- 4 celery stalks
- 1 (1-inch) piece fresh ginger, peeled
- 1 lemon, peeled

Directions:

Add all ingredients into a juicer and extract the juice according to the manufacturer's method.

Pour into 2 glasses and serve immediately.

Lemony Green Juice

Preparation time: 10 minutes   Servings: 2

Ingredients:

- 2 large green apples, cored and sliced
- 4 cups fresh kale leaves
- 4 tablespoons fresh parsley leaves
- 1 tablespoon fresh ginger, peeled
- 1 lemon, peeled
- ½ cup filtered water
- Pinch of salt

Directions:

1. Place all the ingredients in a blender and pulse until well combined.
2. Through a fine mesh strainer, strain the juice and transfer into 2 glasses.
3. Serve immediately.

Kale Scramble

Preparation time: 10 minutes   Cooking time: 6 minutes   Servings: 2

Ingredients:

- 4 eggs
- 1/8 teaspoon ground turmeric
- Salt and ground black pepper, to taste
- 1 tablespoon water
- 2 teaspoons olive oil
- 1 cup fresh kale, tough ribs removed and chopped

Directions:

1. In a bowl, add the eggs, turmeric, salt, black pepper, and water and with a whisk, beat until foamy.
2. In a wok, heat the oil over medium heat.
3. Add the egg mixture and stir to combine.

4. Immediately, reduce the heat to medium-low and cook for about 1–2 minutes, stirring frequently.
5. Stir in the kale and cook for about 3–4 minutes, stirring frequently.
6. Remove from the heat and serve immediately.

Buckwheat Porridge

Preparation time: 10 minutes   Cooking time: 15 minutes   Servings: 2

Ingredients

- 1 cup buckwheat, rinsed
- 1 cup unsweetened almond milk
- 1 cup water
- ½ teaspoon ground cinnamon
- ½ teaspoon vanilla extract
- 1–2 tablespoons raw honey
- ¼ cup fresh blueberries

Directions:

1. In a pan, add all the ingredients (except honey and blueberries) over medium-high heat and bring to a boil.
2. Now, reduce the heat to low and simmer, covered for about 10 minutes.
3. Stir in the honey and remove from the heat.
4. Set aside, covered, for about 5 minutes.
5. With a fork, fluff the mixture, and transfer into serving bowls.
6. Top with blueberries and serve.

Chocolate Granola

Preparation time: 10 minutes   Cooking time: 38 minutes   Servings: 8

Ingredients

- ¼ cup cacao powder
- ¼ cup maple syrup
- 2 tablespoons coconut oil, melted
- ½ teaspoon vanilla extract
- 1/8 teaspoon salt
- 2 cups gluten-free rolled oats
- ¼ cup unsweetened coconut flakes
- 2 tablespoons chia seeds
- 2 tablespoons unsweetened dark chocolate, chopped finely

Directions:

Preheat your oven to 300ºF and line a medium baking sheet with parchment paper.

In a medium pan, add the cacao powder, maple syrup, coconut oil, vanilla extract, and salt, and mix well.

Now, place pan over medium heat and cook for about 2–3 minutes, or until thick and syrupy, stirring continuously.

Remove from the heat and set aside.

In a large bowl, add the oats, coconut, and chia seeds, and mix well.

Add the syrup mixture and mix until well combined.

Transfer the granola mixture onto a prepared baking sheet and spread in an even layer.

Bake for about 35 minutes.

Remove from the oven and set aside for about 1 hour.

Add the chocolate pieces and stir to combine.

Serve immediately.

Blueberry Muffins

Preparation time: 15 minutes   Cooking time: 20 minutes   Servings: 8

Ingredients

- 1 cup buckwheat flour
- ¼ cup arrowroot starch
- 1½ teaspoons baking powder
- ¼ teaspoon sea salt
- 2 eggs
- ½ cup unsweetened almond milk
- 2–3 tablespoons maple syrup
- 2 tablespoons coconut oil, melted
- 1 cup fresh blueberries

Directions:

Preheat your oven to 350ºF and line 8 cups of a muffin tin.

In a bowl, place the buckwheat flour, arrowroot starch, baking powder, and salt, and mix well.

In a separate bowl, place the eggs, almond milk, maple syrup, and coconut oil, and beat until well combined.

Now, place the flour mixture and mix until just combined.

Gently, fold in the blueberries.

Transfer the mixture into prepared muffin cups evenly.

Bake for about 25 minutes or until a toothpick inserted in the center comes out clean.

Remove the muffin tin from oven and place onto a wire rack to cool for about 10 minutes.

Carefully invert the muffins onto the wire rack to cool completely before serving.

Blackcurrant Yogurt Parfait

Ingredients:

- 1 c. natural yogurt (Greek yogurt is acceptable)
- ½ c. blackcurrants
- ½ c. water
- ¼ c. whole oats
- 1 tsp. sugar

Directions:

1. Preheat the oven to 350 degrees.

2. Spread the oats onto a lined cookie sheet and bake until they are lightly golden brown, or about 15 minutes. Allow to cool.

3. In a small pot, combine the blackcurrants and sugar. Bring to a boil and cook for about five minutes, or until the compote thickens. Remove from the heat.

4. In a cup, alternate layers of yogurt, oats, and blackcurrant compote.

5. Garnish with whole blackcurrants and serve immediately.

Shrimp Stir Fry with Buckwheat Noodles

Ingredients:

- 5 oz. shrimp, shelled and deveined
- ½ c. green beans, chopped
- ½ c. kale, roughly chopped
- 1/3 c. celery, chopped
- 1 chili (jalapeño or bird's-eye), chopped and seeded
- ¼ c. chicken stock
- 1 garlic clove, minced
- 1 Tbsp. red onion, chopped
- 2 tsp. soy sauce or tamari
- 2 tsp. olive oil
- 1 tsp. finely chopped fresh ginger
- 1 tsp. lovage or celery leaves, chopped

Directions:

1. In a wok or large skillet, cook the shrimp in one teaspoon of the oil and one teaspoon of the soy sauce or tamari. Cook until they are just opaque, then remove to a place and wipe out the pan.

2. Cook the buckwheat noodles per the package instructions. When they are cooked, drain them and put them in a bowl.

3. Put the remaining oil and soy sauce in the wok or skillet. Add the green beans, kale, celery, chili, red onion, garlic and ginger. Cook until the green beans are crisp-tender, about four to five minutes.

4. Add the shrimp, noodles, and chicken stock to the pan and stir until everything is combined.

5. Remove from heat and serve, sprinkling the lovage or celery leaves over the top.

Aromatic Chicken Salad

Ingredients:

- 4 ounces boneless, skinless chicken breast
- 2 c. baby kale, stems removed
- ½ c. cherry tomatoes
- ¼ c. blueberries
- ¼ c. chopped red onion
- ½ tsp. turmeric
- 1 tsp. light olive oil
- Salt and pepper to taste

Directions:

1. Pound out the chicken breast until it has an even thickness.

2. Sprinkle the chicken with turmeric, salt, and pepper on both sides.

3. Heat the olive oil in a skillet over medium heat.

4. Cook the chicken breast for four minutes, then flip and cook for another three or four minutes or until cooked through. Remove from the pan.

5. In a large bowl, combine the kale, tomatoes, blueberries, and red onions.

6. Slice the chicken and add it to the bowl.

Spinach and Salmon Wraps

Ingredients:

- 4 ounces salmon
- 2 handfuls baby spinach leaves
- 1 handful baby kale, stems removed
- 1 buckwheat wrap
- 2 tsp. light olive oil, divided
- 1 tsp. prepared Dijon mustard.

Directions:

1. Heat one teaspoon of the olive oil in a skillet.

2. Add the salmon and cook until the fish easily releases from the pan. Flip the fish and continue cooking to the desired degree of doneness. Remove to a plate and allow to cool.

3. Spread out the buckwheat wrap and top with the baby spinach and kale.

4. Using a fork, shred the salmon and put it on top of the greens.

5. In a small bowl, whisk together the olive oil and the Dijon mustard until it makes a smooth vinaigrette.

6. Drizzle the vinaigrette over the salmon.

7. Roll the buckwheat wrap carefully, securing with a toothpick.

8. Cut the wrap in half and serve immediately.

Greek Salad Skewers

Ingredients:

- 2 wooden skewers
- 8 large olives, pitted
- 8 cherry tomatoes
- 1 yellow pepper, seeded and cut into 8 pieces
- ½ red onion, cut into 8 pieces
- 8 slices of cucumber
- 8 1-inch cubes of feta cheese
- 1 Tbsp. extra virgin olive oil
- 1 Tbsp. fresh squeezed lemon juice
- 1 tsp. aged balsamic vinegar
- 1 tsp. fresh oregano, chopped
- Salt & pepper to taste

Directions:

1. Thread the ingredients onto the skewers, alternating as follows: olive, tomato, pepper, onion, cucumber, and feta cheese. You should end up with two of each item on each skewer.

2. In a small bowl, combine the olive oil, lemon juice, balsamic vinegar, oregano, salt, and pepper until completely mixed.

3. Drizzle the dressing over the skewers and serve immediately.

Chocolate Waffles

Preparation time: 15 minutes   Cooking time: 24 minutes   Servings: 8

Ingredients

- 2 cups unsweetened almond milk
- 1 tablespoon fresh lemon juice
- 1 cup buckwheat flour
- ½ cup cacao powder
- ¼ cup flaxseed meal
- 1 teaspoon baking soda
- 1 teaspoon baking powder
- ¼ teaspoons kosher salt
- 2 large eggs
- ½ cup coconut oil, melted
- ¼ cup dark brown sugar
- 2 teaspoons vanilla extract
- 2 ounces unsweetened dark chocolate, chopped roughly

Directions:

In a bowl, add the almond milk and lemon juice and mix well.

Set aside for about 10 minutes.

In a bowl, place buckwheat flour, cacao powder, flaxseed meal, baking soda, baking powder, and salt, and mix well.

In the bowl of almond milk mixture, place the eggs, coconut oil, brown sugar, and vanilla extract, and beat until smooth.

Now, place the flour mixture and beat until smooth.

Gently, fold in the chocolate pieces.

Preheat the waffle iron and then grease it.

Place the desired amount of the mixture into the preheated waffle iron and cook for about 3 minutes, or until golden-brown. Repeat with the remaining mixture.

Salmon & Kale Omelet

Preparation time: 10 minutes   Cooking time: 7 minutes   Servings: 4

Ingredients

- 6 eggs
- 2 tablespoons unsweetened almond milk
- Salt and ground black pepper, to taste
- 2 tablespoons olive oil
- 4 ounces smoked salmon, cut into bite-sized chunks
- 2 cup fresh kale, tough ribs removed and chopped finely
- 4 scallions, chopped finely

Directions:

1. In a bowl, place the eggs, coconut milk, salt, and black pepper, and beat well. Set aside.
2. In a non-stick wok, heat the oil over medium heat.
3. Place the egg mixture evenly and cook for about 30 seconds, without stirring.
4. Place the salmon kale and scallions on top of egg mixture evenly.
5. Now, reduce heat to low.
6. With the lid, cover the wok and cook for about 4–5 minutes, or until omelet is done completely.
7. Uncover the wok and cook for about 1 minute.
8. Carefully, transfer the omelet onto a serving plate and serve.

Moroccan Spiced Eggs

Preparation time: 1 hour   Cooking time: 50 minutes   Servings: 2

Ingredients:

- 1 tsp olive oil
- One shallot, stripped and finely hacked
- One red (chime) pepper, deseeded and finely hacked
- One garlic clove, stripped and finely hacked
- One courgette (zucchini), stripped and finely hacked
- 1 tbsp tomato puree (glue)
- ½ tsp gentle stew powder
- ¼ tsp ground cinnamon
- ¼ tsp ground cumin
- ½ tsp salt
- One × 400g (14oz) can hacked tomatoes
- 1 x 400g (14oz) may chickpeas in water
- a little bunch of level leaf parsley (10g (1/3oz)), cleaved
- Four medium eggs at room temperature

Directions:

1. Heat the oil in a pan, include the shallot and red (ringer) pepper and fry delicately for 5 minutes. At that point include the garlic and courgette (zucchini) and cook for one more moment or two. Include the tomato puree (glue), flavours and salt and mix through.
2. Add the cleaved tomatoes and chickpeas (dousing alcohol and all) and increment the warmth to medium. With the top of the dish, stew the sauce for 30 minutes – ensure it is delicately rising all through and permit it to lessen in volume by around 33%.
3. Remove from the warmth and mix in the cleaved parsley.
4. Preheat the grill to 200C/180C fan/350F.

5. When you are prepared to cook the eggs, bring the tomato sauce up to a delicate stew and move to a little broiler confirmation dish.

6. Crack the eggs on the dish and lower them delicately into the stew. Spread with thwart and prepare in the grill for 10-15 minutes. Serve the blend in unique dishes with the eggs coasting on the top.

Chilaquiles with Gochujang

Preparation time: 30 minutes   Cooking time: 20 minutes   Servings: 2

Ingredients:

- One dried ancho chile
- 2 cups of water
- 1 cup squashed tomatoes
- Two cloves of garlic
- One teaspoon genuine salt
- 1/2 tablespoons gochujang
- 5 to 6 cups tortilla chips
- Three enormous eggs
- One tablespoon olive oil

Directions:

1. Get the water to heat a pot. I cheated marginally and heated the water in an electric pot and emptied it into the pan. There's no sound unrivalled strategy here. Add the anchor Chile to the bubbled water and drench for 15 minutes to give it an opportunity to stout up.

2. When completed, use tongs or a spoon to extricate Chile. Make sure to spare the water for the sauce! Nonetheless, on the off chance that you incidentally dump the water, it's not the apocalypse.

3. Mix the doused Chile, 1 cup of saved high temp water, squashed tomatoes, garlic, salt and gochujang until smooth.

4. Empty sauce into a large dish and warmth over medium warmth for 4 to 5 minutes. Mood killer the heat and include the tortilla chips. Mix the chips to

cover with the sauce. In a different skillet, shower a teaspoon of oil and fry an egg on top, until the whites have settled. Plate the egg and cook the remainder of the eggs. If you are phenomenal at performing various tasks, you can likely sear the eggs while you heat the red sauce. I am not precisely so capable.

5. Top the chips with the seared eggs, cotija, hacked cilantro, jalapeños, onions and avocado. Serve right away.

Twice Baked Breakfast Potatoes

Preparation time: 1 hour 10 minutes   Cooking time: 1 hour   Servings: 2

Ingredients:

- 2 medium reddish brown potatoes, cleaned and pricked with a fork everywhere
- 2 tablespoons unsalted spread
- 3 tablespoons overwhelming cream
- 4 rashers cooked bacon
- 4 huge eggs
- ½ cup destroyed cheddar
- Daintily cut chives
- Salt and pepper to taste

Directions:

1. Preheat grill to 400°F.
2. Spot potatoes straightforwardly on stove rack in the focal point of the grill and prepare for 30 to 45 min.
3. Evacuate and permit potatoes to cool for around 15 minutes.
4. Cut every potato down the middle longwise and burrow every half out, scooping the potato substance into a blending bowl.
5. Gather margarine and cream to the potato and pound into a single unit until smooth — season with salt and pepper and mix.

6. Spread a portion of the potato blend into the base of each emptied potato skin and sprinkle with one tablespoon cheddar (you may make them remain pounded potato left to snack on).
7. Add one rasher bacon to every half and top with a raw egg.
8. Spot potatoes onto a heating sheet and come back to the appliance.
9. Lower broiler temperature to 375°F and heat potatoes until egg whites simply set and yolks are as yet runny.
10. Top every potato with a sprinkle of the rest of the cheddar, season with salt and pepper and finish with cut chives.

Sirt Muesli

Preparation time: 30 minutes   Cooking time: 0 minutes   Servings: 2

Ingredients:

- 20g buckwheat drops
- 10g buckwheat puffs
- 15g coconut drops or dried up coconut
- 40g Medjool dates, hollowed and slashed
- 15g pecans, slashed
- 10g cocoa nibs
- 100g strawberries, hulled and slashed
- 100g plain Greek yoghurt (or vegetarian elective, for example, soya or coconut yoghurt)

Directions:

Blend the entirety of the above fixings (forget about the strawberries and yoghurt if not serving straight away).

Mushroom Scramble Eggs

Preparation time: 45 minutes   Cooking time: 10 minutes   Servings: 2

Ingredients:

- 2 eggs
- 1 tsp ground turmeric
- 1 tsp mellow curry powder
- 20g kale, generally slashed
- 1 tsp additional virgin olive oil
- ½ superior bean stew, daintily cut
- bunch of catch mushrooms, meagerly cut
- 5g parsley, finely slashed
- *optional* Add a seed blend as a topper and some Rooster Sauce for enhance

Directions:

1. Blend the turmeric and curry powder and include a little water until you have accomplished a light glue.
2. Steam the kale for 2–3 minutes.
3. Warmth the oil in a skillet over medium heat and fry the bean stew and mushrooms for 2–3 minutes until they have begun to darker and mollify.
4. Include the eggs and flavour glue and cook over a medium warmth at that point add the kale and keep on cooking over medium heat for a further moment. At long last, include the parsley, blend well and serve.

Smoked Salmon Omelets

Preparation time: 45 minutes   Cooking time: 15 minutes   Servings: 2

Ingredients:

- 2 Medium eggs
- 100 g Smoked salmon, cut
- 1/2 tsp Capers
- 10 g Rocket, slashed
- 1 tsp Parsley, slashed
- 1 tsp extra virgin olive oil

Directions:

1. Split the eggs into a bowl and whisk well. Include the salmon, tricks, rocket and parsley.
2. Warmth the olive oil in a non-stick skillet until hot yet not smoking. Include the egg blend and, utilizing a spatula or fish cut, move the mixture around the dish until it is even. Diminish the warmth and let the omelette cook through. Slide the spatula around the edges and move up or crease the omelette fifty-fifty to serve.

Date and Walnut Porridge

Preparation time: 55 minutes   Cooking time: 30 minutes   Servings: 2

Ingredients:

- 200 ml Milk or without dairy elective
- 1 Medjool date, hacked
- 35 g Buckwheat chips
- 1 tsp. Pecan spread or four cleaved pecan parts
- 50 g Strawberries, hulled

Directions:

Spot the milk and time in a dish, heat tenderly, at that point include the buckwheat chips and cook until the porridge is your ideal consistency.

Mix in the pecan margarine or pecans, top with the strawberries and serve.

Shakshuka

Preparation time: 55 minutes   Cooking time: 30 minutes   Servings: 2

Ingredients:

- 1 tsp extra virgin olive oil
- 40g Red onion, finely hacked
- 1 Garlic clove, finely hacked
- 30g Celery, finely hacked
- 1 Bird's eye stew, finely hacked
- 1 tsp ground cumin
- 1 tsp ground turmeric
- 1 tsp Paprika
- 400g Tinned hacked tomatoes
- 30g Kale stems expelled and generally hacked
- 1 tbsp Chopped parsley
- 2 Medium eggs

Directions:

1. Heat a little, profound sided skillet over medium-low warmth. Include the oil and fry the onion, garlic, celery, stew and flavours for 1–2 minutes.
2. Add the tomatoes, at that point, leave the sauce to stew tenderly for 20 minutes, mixing incidentally.
3. Add the kale and cook for a more 5 minutes. If you realize the sauce is getting excessively thick, just include a little water. At the point when your sauce has a pleasant creamy consistency, mix in the parsley.
4. Make two small wells in the sauce and split each egg into them. Decrease the warmth to its most minimal setting and spread the container with a cover or foil. Put the eggs to cook for 10–12 minutes, so, all in all, the whites ought to be firm while the yolks are as yet runny. Cook a further 3–4 minutes if you lean toward the eggs to be firm. Serve promptly – in a perfect world directly from the skillet.

Moroccan Spiced Eggs

Preparation time: 1 hour 10 minutes   Cooking time: 45 minutes   Servings: 2

Ingredients:

- 1 tsp olive oil
- One shallot, stripped and finely hacked
- One red (chime) pepper, deseeded and finely hacked
- One garlic clove, stripped and finely hacked
- One courgette (zucchini), stripped and finely hacked
- 1 tbsp tomato puree (glue)
- ½ tsp gentle stew powder
- ¼ tsp ground cinnamon
- One × 400g (14oz) can hacked tomatoes
- 1 x 400g (14oz) may chickpeas in water
- a little bunch of level leaf parsley (10g (1/3oz)), cleaved
- Four medium eggs at room temperature
- ¼ tsp ground cumin
- ½ tsp salt

Directions:

1. Heat the oil in a pan, include the shallot and red (ringer) pepper and fry delicately for 5 minutes. At that point include the garlic and courgette (zucchini) and cook for one more moment or two. Include the tomato puree (glue), flavours and salt and mix through.
2. Add the cleaved tomatoes and chickpeas (dousing alcohol and all) and increment the warmth to medium. With the top of the dish, stew the sauce for 30 minutes – ensure it is delicately rising all through and permit it to lessen in volume by around 33%.
3. Remove from the warmth and mix in the cleaved parsley.
4. Preheat the grill to 200C/180C fan/350F.
5. When you are prepared to cook the eggs, bring the tomato sauce up to a delicate stew and move to a little broiler confirmation dish.
6. Crack the eggs on the dish and lower them delicately into the stew. Spread with thwart and prepare in the grill for 10-15 minutes. Serve the blend in unique dishes with the eggs coasting on the top.

Mushroom Dinner Scramble

Ingredients:

- 2 medium eggs at room temperature
- 1 handful baby kale, chopped
- ½ c. white button mushrooms, sliced
- ½ jalapeño pepper, seeded and chopped
- 1 Tbsp. flat leaf parsley, chopped
- 1 tsp. ground turmeric
- 1 tsp. mild curry powder
- 1 tsp. olive oil

Directions:

1. In a small dish, combine the turmeric and curry powder with a little water and stir until it makes a paste.

2. Heat the olive oil in a skillet over medium-high heat.

3. Add the mushrooms, jalapeno, and turmeric-curry paste, and cook over medium heat until the mushrooms have softened and browned.

4. In a small bowl, beat the eggs. Pour them over the mushrooms and chilies.

5. Using a rubber spatula or wooden spoon, gently scramble the eggs as they cook.

6. Just before the eggs are done, add the kale and parsley, stirring to allow the heat of the eggs to wilt the greens.

7. Serve immediately. If you wish, you can serve this with lettuce leaves for wrapping, or with a buckwheat wrap.

Marinated Cod and Asparagus

Ingredients:

- 5 ounces black cod or Atlantic cod
- 4 teaspoons miso paste
- 1 Tbsp. mirin
- 1 Tbsp. extra virgin olive oil, divided
- 8 ounces asparagus
- 1 tsp. soy sauce or tamari
- 1 tsp. sesame seeds

Directions:

1. Preheat the oven to 350 degrees.

2. In a small bowl, mix the miso, mirin, and one teaspoon of the olive oil. Pour the marinade over the cod and allow it to marinate for at least 30 minutes.

3. Mix one teaspoon of the olive oil with the soy sauce and pour over the asparagus. Transfer the asparagus to a lined cookie sheet or a shallow baking dish. Bake the asparagus until it just begins to brown, about 25 to 30 minutes.

4. In a skillet, heat the remaining one teaspoon of the olive oil. Remove the cod from the marinade and add it to the pan, reserving the marinade. Cook it for five minutes or until the fish separates easily from the pan and can be flipped. Turn it and continue cooking until the fish is opaque and flaky.

5. Remove the fish and add the marinade to the pan. Cook until the marinade boils, then lower the heat and continue cooking until the marinade is reduced by half.

6. Serve the cod with a drizzle of the cooked-down marinade and a sprinkle of sesame seeds. Serve the asparagus on the side.

Crispy Pork and Tofu Stir Fry

Ingredients:

- 8 ounces extra-firm tofu
- 8 ounces minced pork
- 4 ounces Shiitake mushrooms, sliced
- 4 ounces bok choy, shredded
- 4 ounces bean sprouts
- 2 Tbsp. olive oil

Ingredients for Sauce:

- 4 ounces low-sodium chicken stock
- 1 Tbsp. rice wine
- 1 Tbsp. soy sauce or tamari
- 1 Tbsp. brown sugar
- 1 Tbsp. tomato puree
- 1 Tbsp. corn flour
- 1 Tbsp. water
- 1 Tbsp. ginger, peeled and minced
- 1 clove of garlic, peeled and minced

Directions:

1. Combine the corn flour and water in a small bowl and whisk until it is combined and there are no lumps.

2. Add the remaining sauce ingredients, and stir until combined.

3. Dice the tofu and pat it dry between two layers of paper towel. Allow it to sit on the paper towel until you are ready to use it.

4. Heat the olive oil in a wok. Add the Shiitake mushrooms and cook until they are brown and have begun to soften, about three minutes.

5. Remove the mushrooms and add the tofu and stir fry until it is golden brown on all sides.

6. Remove the tofu and add the bok choy and bean sprouts. Cook until just tender, then add the sauce. Add the mince and tofu back to the wok and stir to coat with the sauce. Continue cooking until just heated through. Serve immediately.

White Bean Stew

Ingredients:

- 8 ounces canned white beans, drained and rinsed
- 8 ounces low-sodium chicken stock
- 1 16-ounce can of chopped tomatoes
- 2 handfuls baby kale, stems removed
- ¼ c. buckwheat
- ½ red onion, finely chopped
- 1 stalk celery, chopped
- 1 carrot, chopped
- 1 garlic clove, minced
- 1 Tbsp. flat leaf parsley, chopped
- 1 Tbsp. extra virgin olive oil
- 1 tsp. tomato puree
- 1 tsp. Herbes de Provence

Directions:

1. Place a large pot over medium heat and heat the olive oil.

2. Add the onion, celery, carrot, and garlic, and herbes de Provence, and cook them until they begin to soften.

3. Add the chicken stock, canned tomatoes, and tomato puree and bring to a boil.

4. Add the beans and simmer for about 30 minutes.

5. Separately, cook the buckwheat according to the package instructions. Drain it and set it aside.

6. Add the kale to the stew and cook until tender, about five to ten minutes.

7. Stir in the parsley at the last minute.

8. Serve the stew with the buckwheat.

Turkey Cutlets with Cauliflower "Risotto"

Ingredients:

- 6 ounces turkey cutlets
- 6 ounces cauliflower
- ½ red onion, chopped
- 1/3 c. sundried tomatoes, chopped
- 1 garlic clove, minced
- ½ lemon, juiced
- 2 Tbsp. extra virgin olive oil
- 1 Tbsp. parsley, chopped
- 1 Tbsp. capers
- 1 Tbsp. fresh ginger, chopped
- 2 tsp. ground turmeric
- 1 tsp. dried sage
- Salt and pepper to taste

Directions:

1. Cut the cauliflower into florets and put it in a food processor, pulsing it until it resembles couscous.

2. Heat one teaspoon of the olive oil in a skillet. Cook the red onion, garlic, and ginger for a minute to release the aromas, then add the cauliflower and turmeric.

3. Cook the cauliflower for 2 minutes, or until just softened. Remove it from the heat and stir in the sundried tomatoes and parsley.

4. Heat the remaining olive oil in a large skillet. Sprinkle the turkey cutlets with the dried sage, salt, and pepper. Cook the cutlets for two minutes on each side or until just cooked through.

5. Remove the turkey from the pan and add the lemon juice and capers, scraping to deglaze the pan. Continue to cook until the liquid reduces a bit.

6. Slice the turkey and serve it over the "couscous" with a drizzle of the sauce.

Baked Salmon Salad with Creamy Mint Dressing

Preparation time: 55 minutes   Cooking time: 20 minutes   Serving: 1

Ingredients

- 1 salmon fillet (130g)
- 40g mixed salad leaves
- 40g young spinach leaves
- 2 radishes, trimmed and thinly sliced
- 5cm piece (50g) cucumber, cut into chunks
- 2 spring onions, trimmed and sliced
- one small handful (10g) parsley, roughly chopped

For the dressing

- 1 tsp low-fat mayonnaise
- 1 tbsp natural yoghurt
- 1 tbsp rice vinegar
- 2 leaves mint, finely chopped
- Salt to taste
- Freshly ground black pepper

Directions:

1. First, preheat your oven to 200°C
2. (180°C fan/Gas 6).
3. Now place the salmon fillet on a baking tray. Bake it for 16–18 minutes until cooked. Now remove it from the oven and set aside. The salmon is equally useful to be you used as hot or cold in the salad. If salmon has skin, simply cook skin side down. Remove the salmon from the skin. It slides off easily when cooked.
4. Now mix the mayonnaise, yoghurt, rice wine vinegar, and the mint leaves. Add salt and pepper.
5. Leave them to stand for at least 5 minutes. It allows the flavours to develop.

6. Arrange salad leaves and spinach on a serving plate. Top with the radishes, cucumber, the spring onions and parsley. Now Flake the cooked salmon onto the salad. Finally, drizzle the dressing over.

Coronation Chicken Salad

Preparation time: 5 minutes   Cooking time: 0 minutes   Servings: 1

Ingredients

- 75 g Natural yoghurt
- Juice of 1/4 of a lemon
- 1 tsp Coriander, chopped
- 1 tsp ground turmeric
- 1/2 tsp Mild curry powder
- 100 g Cooked chicken breast, cut into bite-sized pieces
- 6 Walnut halves, finely chopped
- 1 Medjool date, finely chopped
- 20 g Red onion, diced
- 1 Bird's eye chilli
- 40 g Rocket (for serving)

Directions:

Mix the yoghurt, lemon juice, coriander and the spices. Add all the remaining ingredients now. Serve on a bed of the rocket.

Baked Potatoes with Spicy Chickpea Stew

Preparation time: 10 minutes   Cooking time: 1 hour   Servings: 4-6

Ingredients

- 4-6 baking potatoes, pricked all over
- 2 tablespoons olive oil
- 2 red onions, finely chopped
- 4 cloves garlic, grated or crushed
- 2cm ginger, grated
- ½ -2 teaspoons chilli flakes (depending on how hot you like things)
- 2 tablespoons cumin seeds
- 2 tablespoons turmeric
- Splash of water
- 2 x 400g tins chopped tomatoes
- 2 tablespoons unsweetened cocoa powder (or cacao)
- 2 x 400g tins chickpeas (or kidney beans if you prefer) including the chickpea water DON'T DRAIN!!
- 2 yellow peppers (or whatever colour you prefer!), chopped into bite size pieces
- 2 tablespoons parsley plus extra for garnish
- Salt and pepper to taste (optional)
- Side salad

Directions:

1. Preheat the oven to 200C.
2. Meanwhile prepare all the other ingredients.
3. When the oven is hot enough, then put your baking potatoes in the oven. Cook for 1 hour.
4. Once the potatoes are in the oven, then place the olive oil and chopped red onion in a large wide saucepan. Cook it gently, with the lid on for 5 minutes. Continue cooking until the onions are soft but not brown.

5. Remove the lid. Add the garlic, ginger, cumin and chilli. Now cook for a minute on low heat. Then add the turmeric and a tiny splash of water and cook for one minute. Take care that pan does get too dry.

6. Now add in the tomatoes, cocoa powder (or cacao), chickpeas (also include the chickpea water). Also, add yellow pepper and bring to boil. Simmer on a low heat for about 45 minutes. Hence the sauce is thick (but don't let it burn!).

7. The stew should be cooked roughly at the same time as the potatoes.

8. Finally, stir in the two tablespoons of parsley, and some salt and pepper if you wish. Finally, serve the stew on top of the baked potatoes.

Chargrilled Beef with a Red Wine Jus, Onion Rings, Garlic Kale& Herb-Roasted Potatoes

Preparation time: Cooking time: Servings: 2

Ingredients

- 100 grams potatoes (peeled and cut into 2cm dice)
- 1 tbsp extra virgin olive oil
- 5g parsley, finely chopped
- 50g red onion, sliced into rings
- 50g Kale, sliced
- 1 garlic clove, finely chopped
- 120–150g x 3.5cm-thick beef fillet steak or 2cm-thick sirloin steak
- 40ml red wine
- 150ml beef stock
- 1 tsp tomato purée
- 1 tsp corn flour, dissolved in 1 tbsp water

Directions:

Heat your oven to 220ºC/gas 7.

Place the potatoes in a saucepan with boiling water.

Bring back to the boil now cook for 4–5 minutes.

108

Drain.

Now place in a roasting tin with 1 teaspoon of the oil. Roast it in the hot oven for about 35 to 45 mins.

Turn the potatoes every 10 minutes.

When it is cooked, remove from the oven. Then sprinkle with the chopped parsley and mix well.

Fry the onion in 1 teaspoon oil and heat for 5 minutes. Fry till they get soft and nicely caramelized. Keep warm. Now steam the Kale for 2–3 minutes then drain.

Fry the garlic gently oil (1/2 tablespoon oil). Fry for one minute. It should get soft, but it should not be coloured. Add the Kale and fry for 2 minutes more, until it gets tender. Keep warm.

Heat a frying pan over high heat. Heat until smoking.

Coat the meat in ½ teaspoon of the oil, fry in the hot pan over a medium to high temperature, i.e. heat according to how you like your meat cooked.

If you like to cook the meat on a medium level, it would be better to sear the meat. Now transfer the pan to an oven set at 220ºC/gas 7. Finish the cooking that way for a specific time.

Remove the meat from the pan. Set aside to rest. Now add the wine to the hot pan to bring up if any meat residue is left. Bubble to reduce the wine by its half. It becomes syrupy with a thick flavour in this way.

Add stock and tomato purée to the steak pan to boil it. Then keep adding the corn flour paste to thicken the sauce, adding it a little at a time until you have your desired thickness.

Stir in any of the juices from your steak.

Serve it with the roasted potatoes, Kale, onion rings and the red wine sauce.

Buckwheat Pasta Salad

Preparation time: 30 minutes   Cooking time: 0 minutes   Servings 1

Ingredients

- 50g buckwheat pasta
- large handful of rocket
- a small handful of basil leaves
- 8 cherry tomatoes, halved
- 1/2 avocado, diced
- 10 olives
- 1 tbsp extra virgin olive oil
- 20g pine nuts

Directions:

Combine all the ingredients. Don't include the pine nuts. Arrange on a plate. Scatter the pine nuts over the top.

Greek Salad Skewers

Preparation time: 45 minutes   Cooking time: 10 minutes   Servings: 2

Ingredients:

- 2 wooden skewers, soaked in water for 30 minutes before use
- 8 large black olives
- 8 cherry tomatoes
- 1 yellow pepper, cut into eight squares
- ½ red onion, chopped in half and separated into eight pieces
- 100g (about 10cm) cucumber, cut into four slices and halved
- 100g feta, cut into 8 cubes

For the dressing

- 1 tbsp extra virgin olive oil
- Juice of ½ lemon
- 1 tsp balsamic vinegar

- ½ clove garlic, peeled and crushed
- Few leaves of basil, finely chopped (or ½ tsp dried mixed herbs to replace basil and oregano)
- Few leaves oregano (finely chopped)
- generous seasoning of salt and ground black pepper

Directions:

First of all thread each skewer with the salad ingredients in the following order: - Olive, Tomato, Yellow pepper, Red onion, Cucumber, Feta, Tomato, Olive, Yellow pepper, Red onion, Cucumber, and Feta.

Now place all the dressing ingredients in a small bowl. Mix together and pour over the skewers.

Kale, Edamame and Tofu Curry

Preparation time: 1 hour   Cooking time: 45 minutes   Servings: 4

Ingredients:

- 1 tbsp rapeseed oil
- 1 large onion, chopped
- 4 cloves garlic, peeled and grated
- 4 .1 large thumb (7cm) fresh ginger, peeled and grated
- 1 red chilli, deseeded and thinly sliced
- 1/2 tsp ground turmeric
- 1/4 tsp cayenne pepper
- 1 tsp paprika
- 1/2 tsp ground cumin
- 1 tsp salt
- 250g dried red lentils
- 1 litre boiling water
- 50g frozen soyaedamame beans
- 200g firm tofu, chopped into cubes
- 2 tomatoes, roughly chopped

- Juice of 1 lime
- 200g kale leaves, stalks removed and torn

Directions:

1. Put the oil in a heavy-bottomed pan. Cook over low to medium heat. Add the onion in it and cook for 5 minutes.
2. Then add the garlic, ginger and chilli. After adding them and cook for two minutes.
3. Add turmeric, cayenne, paprika, cumin and salt. Stir through before you add the red lentils. Stir again.
4. Pour in the boiling water. Boil for 10 minutes. Now reduce the heat and cook for a further 20-30 minutes until the curry has a thick '•porridge' consistency.
5. Add the soya beans, tofu and tomatoes, cook for 5 minutes more. Add the lime juice and kale leaves. Cook until the Kale is just tender.

Sirt Food Miso-Marinated Cod with Stir-Fried Greens and Sesame

Preparation time: 1 hour 10 minutes   Cooking time: 40 minutes   Servings: 1

Ingredients

- 20g miso
- 1 tbsp mirin
- 1 tbsp extra virgin olive oil
- 200g skinless cod fillet
- 20g red onion, sliced
- 40g celery, sliced
- one garlic clove, finely chopped
- one bird's eye chilli, finely chopped
- 1 tsp finely chopped fresh ginger
- 60g green beans
- 50g Kale, roughly chopped
- 1 tsp sesame seeds

- 5g parsley, roughly chopped
- 1 tbsp tamari
- 30g buckwheat
- 1 tsp ground turmeric

Directions:

1. Mix the miso and mirin with one teaspoon of the oil.
2. Rub all over cod and leave to marinate. Marinate for 30 minutes. Now heat the oven to 220ºC/gas 7. Bake the cod for 10 minutes. Next heat a frying pan or wok with the remaining oil.
3. Add the onion to it and stir-fry for a few minutes. Add celery, garlic, chilli, ginger, green beans and Kale, all of them. Toss and fry until the Kale is tender and is cooked well, add a little water to the pan to aid the cooking process.
4. Cook the buckwheat according to the instructions on the packet. Cook it with turmeric for three minutes. Now add the sesame seeds, parsley and tamari to the stir-fry. Serve it with the greens and fish.

Chocolate Bark

Preparation time: 30 minutes   Cooking time: 3 hours   Servings: 2

Ingredients:

- 1 thin peel orange
- ¾ cup pistachio nuts, roasted, chilled and chopped into large pieces
- ¼ cup hazelnuts, toasted, chilled, peeled and chopped into large pieces
- ¼ cup pumpkin seeds, toasted and chilled
- 1 tablespoon chia seeds
- 1 tablespoon sesame seeds, toasted and cooled
- 1 teaspoon grated orange peel
- 1 cardamom pod, finely crushed and sieved
- 12 ounces (340 g) tempered, dairy-free dark chocolate (65% cocoa content)
- 2 teaspoons flaky sea salt
- Candy or candy thermometer

Directions:

1. Preheat the oven to 100-150 ° F (66 ° C). Line a baking sheet with parchment paper.

2. Finely slice the orange crosswise and place it on the prepared baking sheet. Bake for 2 to 3 hours until dry but slightly sticky. Remove it from the oven and let it cool.

3. When they cool enough to handle them, cut the orange slices into fragments; set them aside.

4. In a large bowl, mix the nuts, seeds, and grated orange peel until completely combined. Place the mixture in a single layer on a baking sheet lined with kitchen parchment. Set it aside.

5. Melt the chocolate in a water bath until it reaches 88 to 90 ° F (32 to 33 ° C) and pours it over the nut mixture to cover it completely.

6. When the chocolate is semi-cold but still sticky, sprinkle the surface with sea salt and pieces of orange.

7. Place the mixture in a cold area of your kitchen or refrigerate until the crust cools completely, and cut it into bite-sized pieces.

Salmon and Spinach Quiche

Preparation time: 55 minutes   Cooking time: 45 minutes   Servings: 2

Ingredients:

- 600 g frozen leaf spinach
- 1 clove of garlic
- 1 onion
- 150 g frozen salmon fillets
- 200 g smoked salmon
- 1 small Bunch of dill
- 1 untreated lemon
- 50 g butter
- 200 g sour cream
- 3 eggs
- Salt, pepper, nutmeg
- 1 pack of puff pastry

Directions:

1. Let the spinach thaw and squeeze well.
2. Peel the garlic and onion and cut into fine cubes.
3. Cut the salmon fillet into cubes 1-1.5 cm thick.
4. Cut the smoked salmon into strips.
5. Wash the dill, pat dry and chop.
6. Wash the lemon with hot water, dry, rub the zest finely with a kitchen grater and squeeze the lemon.
7. Heat the butter in a pan. Sweat the garlic and onion cubes in it for approx. 2-3 minutes.
8. Add spinach and sweat briefly.
9. Add sour cream, lemon juice and zest, eggs and dill and mix well.
10. Season with salt, pepper and nutmeg.
11. Preheat the oven to 200 degrees top / bottom heat (180 degrees convection).
12. Grease a springform pan and roll out the puff pastry in it and pull up on edge. Prick the dough with a fork (so that it doesn't rise too much).
13. Pour in the spinach and egg mixture and smooth out.
14. Spread salmon cubes and smoked salmon strips on top.
15. The quiche in the oven (grid, middle inset) about 30-40 min. Yellow gold bake.